MW00640167

* * *

"This is a must-read for caregivers, in what is almost always a difficult, meaningful, or confusing time. *Stand By Me* is a perfect mix of caregiver memoir, love letter, how-to guide, self-help book, and policy treatise on the US's approach to caregiving and workplace policies that facilitate care all wrapped into one. It will help caregivers feel less alone and more empowered in their own caregiving relationship, in their interaction with the healthcare system, and as advocates for a different national approach to work, family, and care."

—Vicki Shabo, senior fellow, New America

* * *

"In combining powerful storytelling with practical tools and strategies, Dr. Applebaum has highlighted the issue of caregiver burden while providing us with a sustainable way forward. *Stand By Me* is a treasure for caregivers, their care recipients and supporters, and the rest of us who will someday need this book."

—Jessica Zitter, MD, MPH, founder of Reel Medicine Media

* * *

"Thoughtful, sensitive, highly practical, easy to read, and based in personal and professional experience, *Stand By Me* is a book to be put to use by family caregivers and one that will also help them in their quest for meaning to keep them going."

—Arthur Kleinman, author of *The Soul of Care*

PRAISE FOR
STAND BY ME

"Weaving her rich personal experience as a caregiver with her role as a national and international expert on caregiving and caregiver support, Dr. Applebaum fuses her personal and professional knowledge in an engaging narrative to speak directly to caregivers. She focuses on the challenges caregivers face in having a voice, feeling alone, and finding meaning in their work as they try to do their best in new roles and responsibilities.

Like a master clinician, Dr. Applebaum supportively defines necessary skills for caregivers and how to learn them, emphasizes the critical need for self-care for the caregiver, and describes what psychological supports are available to help caregivers find meaning in a role that is often frightening, lonely, and unwanted.

Using a range of methods to engage the reader, like checklists and self-questionnaires, Dr. Applebaum encourages caregivers to reflect on their challenges, respond to questions about their roles, responsibilities, and concerns, and to be aware of the resources available to help address these daunting issues. Reading this book is like attending a caregiver clinical consultation offering support, advice, compassion, and competence.

Stand By Me is a rich resource of invaluable information and expert advice for caregivers written by a caregiver and expert psychologist. It needs to be read by caregivers and all healthcare professionals as they struggle to make caregivers collaborators on the healthcare team."

—Dr. Kathleen M. Foley, emeritus member at Memorial Sloan
Kettering Cancer Center and emeritus professor
of neurology at Weill Cornell Medicine

* * *

"*Stand By Me*, first and foremost, is a book about the love between a daughter and a father navigating the challenges of illness and loss. It contains deep wisdom and guidance, offering comfort to those entering into the realm of caregiving. With kindness, humanity, and the insight of someone who knows about being a family caregiver, personally and professionally, Dr. Applebaum shows us how we can stand by and care for the people in our lives who matter during their time of need."

—Dr. Harvey Max Chochinov, distinguished professor of psychiatry at the University of Manitoba and author of *Dignity in Care: The Human Side of Medicine*

* * *

"Warm, compassionate, and brimming with wisdom and expert advice born of the author's deep personal and professional experience, *Stand By Me* sets the new gold standard for caregiving guides. This book is an indispensable read for anyone whose life is touched by caregiving—which is everyone."

—Kate Washington, author of *Already Toast: Caregiving and Burnout in America*

* * *

"*Stand By Me* is a powerful and insightful look into the realities of family caregiving in America. Dr. Applebaum blends her lived experience with deep professional expertise to offer a practical framework for navigating the challenges that shape caregiving, making the physical and emotional work of caregiving more sustainable."

—Jason Resendez, president and CEO, National Alliance for Caregiving

STAND BY ME

A GUIDE TO NAVIGATING MODERN, MEANINGFUL CAREGIVING

Allison J. Applebaum, PhD

SIMON ELEMENT

New York London Toronto Sydney New Delhi

**SIMON
ELEMENT**

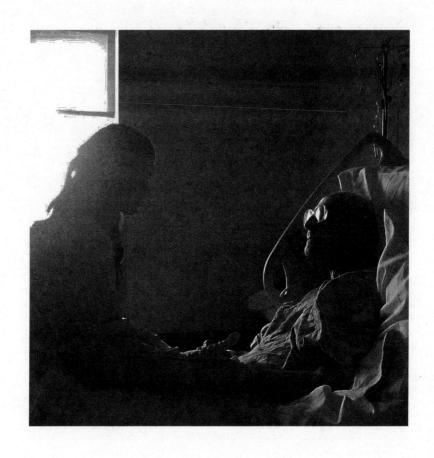

For my father, Stanley S. Applebaum.

CONTENTS

*Chapter subtitles are each the titles of songs composed,
arranged, performed, produced, and/or conducted
by Stanley Applebaum.*

AUTHOR'S NOTE

Confidentiality is at the heart of the therapeutic relationship. Clinical cases presented use pseudonyms and de-identified material and have been altered to protect patients' privacy. In all cases, examples are not based on specific patients but instead represent the collective experiences of caregivers seen in the Caregivers Clinic at Memorial Sloan Kettering Cancer Center.

While cases presented in the following chapters are those of caregivers of patients with cancer, this is not a book written only for caregivers of patients with cancer. Instead, this is a book written to support and honor caregivers of patients with *all* chronic and life-limiting illnesses, conditions, and disabilities.

Finally, while all of the clinical cases presented have been de-identified, I am sharing personal elements of my and my dad's experience as partners in care. Long before his death, my dad and I spoke about this book, and he gave his full consent for me to share our story.

A NOTE ON LANGUAGE

Words matter. The language we use to describe the human experience is essential to understanding individuals' lived experiences. Throughout this book, I use several different words and phrases to refer to caregivers: family and friend caregivers, care partners, partners in care, and simply *caregivers*. I make a point to use these words because they encapsulate what it is that caregivers do: they give of themselves, and they partner with others in care. I am purposefully not using the word *caretaker* or the phrase *informal caregiver* anywhere in this book, as these are inaccurate and misrepresent the intense efforts carried out by caregivers. All of us were, are, or will be caregivers, often repeatedly throughout our lives. And so, all of us know that our caregiving journeys—for ill or disabled family members, for children, for anyone in our lives—are anything but informal.

Throughout, I also use the phrase *loved one* to refer to patients, since this is a phrase used by many caregivers to describe their care partner. However, not all caregivers feel that their partner in care is a loved one. As you read, I encourage you to reflect on what language makes the most sense to you, and if it's different than what I have written, to adopt and insert that word or phrase throughout.

STAND BY ME

PRELUDE

The Causality Dilemma of Caregiving

Allison's Theme

Artist: Stan Applebaum and His Orchestra, 1963

321 days. 7,704 hours. 462,240 minutes. Almost an entire calendar year. Enough time to create a new human. To circle the globe slowly. To take 5,136 ballet classes. To listen to a Rachmaninoff concerto about 15,408 times. Or rather, the rough estimate of the time I spent by my dad's side in emergency departments and hospital rooms. Hours, days, and weeks spent standing by him, serving as his eyes, ears, and often, voice while he lay on stretchers, frequently for days in cold hospital hallways waiting for an inpatient bed to open. Time spent keeping a constant eye out for the signs of delirium in him while I combated what occasionally felt like my own fatigue-induced hallucinations. Months spent with little sense of the change in seasons and weeks where days and nights melded to one. Sometimes the clock ticked so slowly, though later it ticked much, much too fast. This is just a snapshot into the decade I spent by his side, taking care of him, doing what I and others in the field have called serving as his family caregiver, but much more accurately and to the point personally, spent loving him.

My dad, the focus of my caregiving journey, was Stanley Applebaum, the world-renowned composer, orchestrator, and arranger who is perhaps best known for his arrangement for Ben E. King's "Stand By Me." The memorable string line in the middle of "Stand By Me" that gives the song its orchestral feel was my dad's creation, as were hundreds of other arrangements he did for all of the top artists of the 1950s and 1960s. My dad was almost sixty when I came into the picture in November of 1981, and this fact dramatically shaped my life. I feared his death from the day I learned that he was seventy when I was ten, and this fear ultimately inspired within me a drive to live each moment with him as fully as possible. What resulted was the most intensely loving, supportive, and honest relationship I could imagine unfolding between a father and daughter. I treasured every moment we had: from sitting by his side in the car as a child, the car being his classroom for vulnerability and where I learned to embrace authenticity; to sitting together looking out onto the ocean, where he taught me the power of transcendence through nature; to sitting by his side at the piano while we played duets, where he taught me what it means to be a partner; to sitting by his hospital bed, where he taught me the deepest meaning of love. In every sense of the word, he *cared* for me throughout my life, as I did for him until he took his last breath.

Today, the relationship we cultivated inspires me to share our experiences as partners in care, to honor his legacy, and to use our story to support as many caregiving families as possible.

* * *

As a child, I didn't dream of working in healthcare in any way; I certainly never imagined serving as my dad's caregiver and subsequently devoting my life's work to supporting family caregivers. Inspired by my parents' successful artistic careers, by the time I was five I was set on becoming a professional ballet dancer. While friends of mine from school were having playdates in the afternoon, I was going on auditions. At age seven, I made my debut at City Center in New York City in a production of *Cinderella* staged by the Fort Worth Ballet. This was followed by years of intensive training with the Joffrey Ballet in New York City and then the Boston Ballet. This artistic path ended, however, as the towers in lower Manhattan fell on September 11, 2001. I lived close by, and after the second tower collapsed, I ran with other survivors uptown, eventually showing up at my parents' apartment completely emotionally numb. Two days later, I found myself doing what had always brought me a sense of normalcy and grounding: I took a ballet class at Steps on Broadway on the Upper West Side. The reality of what had just happened to our world sunk in, as did the fragility of life. I remember thinking while doing a port de bras at the barre, "There must be more. I need to do more." A few months later I traded in intensive ballet training for a research assistant position in the Department of Psychiatry at Mount Sinai Hospital in New York.

When I began working toward my doctorate in Clinical Psychology at Boston University three years later, my classmates and I joked about doing "Me-search." That is, academic research on a topic of interest to the researcher because of personal connectedness to the issue. For example, some graduate students who have survived eating disorders eventually study the etiology of eating disorders and the psychopathology that maintains these behaviors. Others who are survivors of trauma may devote their careers to the study of post-traumatic stress disorder. Frequently, these choices in academic pursuits are consciously, purposefully made. They provide a way to understand and find benefit from one's past experiences.

I didn't set out to do Me-search; that was never my intention. When I began my postdoctoral fellowship at Memorial Sloan Kettering Cancer Center in 2010 in psycho-oncology—the specialized field that addresses the psychological, behavioral, emotional, and social issues that arise for patients with cancer and their loved ones—I did not identify with the caregiver role. Although my dad was starting to exhibit signs of minor heart and kidney failure and had several hospitalizations between 2010 and 2013, he recovered well from each and was able to return to a full life at home with my mom, composing music and spending nights in the recording studio. At that time, my energy was focused on wrapping up my doctoral studies, transitioning to life back in New York, beginning my career, and trying to have what social life I could in the minimal free time available.

In my first year of fellowship, I provided clinical care to patients with advanced, life-limiting cancers who were facing their last months and weeks of life. This work focused on helping these patients connect to a sense of meaning and purpose in life despite the profound limitations they were facing. Providing this type of care was equally meaningful and purpose-driven for me. That year, I was encouraged to think about what services were needed in the hospital, and more broadly, what areas the field of psycho-oncology had not yet fully addressed. I thought about each time I would accompany a patient with advanced cancer back to a therapy room, leaving their parent, or partner, or child, or sibling, or friend in the waiting room. I thought about how inevitably the chitchat we'd engage in during that walk would center on the person left in the waiting room. I thought about how, in those sessions, one of the most frequent and prominent themes that would emerge was concern about how that parent, or partner, or child, or sibling, or friend was currently doing emotionally, and how they would cope with the patient's eventual death. I thought about how that parent, or partner, or child, or sibling, or friend was in so many ways the linchpin of that patient's care and illness experience, about how the presence and well-being of that parent, or partner, or child, or sibling, or friend would dramatically impact the quality of care that patient would receive. And I thought about the theme that was beginning to emerge in my own therapy appointments in which I was the patient: concern about my dad's growing list of medical problems, my ability to navigate taking care of him, and how I would cope with his eventual death.

It was evident that these parents, partners, children, siblings, and friends of patients receiving medical care, these caregivers, were in desperate need of their own support. In fact, they were worthy and deserving of that support. And so, a year later in 2011, I founded the Caregivers Clinic, the first dedicated clinical service for caregivers in any comprehensive cancer center in this country.[1] The clinic provides support to caregivers of patients with all sites and stages of cancer, across the entire caregiving trajectory, from diagnosis through bereavement. Within the first twelve months of the clinic's opening, there was already a significant waitlist for care; the demand for support for caregivers was immediately evident. That year, I worked with colleagues with expertise in family therapy and bereavement care to envision a program that would provide comprehensive care to families facing cancer. I explored what was being done at cancer centers across the United States to learn more about what was available nationally to support caregivers and began advocating for attention to this issue. And I secured funding from the American Cancer Society to begin a program of research focused on identifying the unique psychosocial needs of cancer caregivers and developing therapeutic interventions that would address those needs. The importance of a targeted service to support caregivers was clear, and in 2013, I joined the faculty of the Department of Psychiatry and Behavioral Sciences as the director of the Caregivers Clinic.

That same year, my own caregiving journey began. My professional identity had already been marked in at least semipermanent ink and the trajectory for my clinical and research activities established. I was not doing Me-search in 2013 but instead the reverse: I had to now experience exactly what I had already sought out to study. For years, I found myself supporting caregivers who were facing similar challenges to those I was confronting outside of work, hearing about navigating the complexities of our healthcare system while I, too, was doing the same. While close colleagues were aware of my caregiving role, the parallel between my work and professional life was something I rarely shared with my broader professional network and never shared with my patients. For many reasons, the therapeutic relationship is often assisted by the relative anonymity of the therapist and self-disclosure on the part of therapists may not necessarily benefit patients. I don't believe it would have been productive for my patients to know about my personal caregiving journey at that time, and I imagined many ways in which disclosing my caregiving status could have impeded the therapeutic processes occurring. Certainly, however, my own experiences allowed me to be intensely empathic and understanding of their challenges, from their sense of isolation and inability to plan for the future, to their concerns about their ability to handle the financial demands of caregiving, to their fear of the death of their loved ones.

My caregiving responsibilities intensified dramatically in 2014. While I had spent the prior two decades anticipating my dad's death, due to a significant age difference between them, I imagined sharing a long future with my mom. My mom was a pianist, singer, performer, and all-around creative genius. Like my dad, she had an incredibly prolific career, concertized around the world, and wrote music for stage and screen. Sadly, that vision of her presence during the unfolding of my adulthood never became a reality; my mom died suddenly in 2014. As I assumed the responsibilities of overseeing all aspects of my dad's care, I stepped into a new phase of caregiving superimposed upon an emotional storm of grief and shock and devastation. It was—and I hope it will remain—the most challenging era of my life.

Inevitably, these deeply personal experiences impacted the questions I was exploring in my research, my approach to patient care, and how I was viewing my professional work. For example, in 2013 my dad was diagnosed with Lewy body disease, a progressive neurodegenerative disease that can lead to problems with thinking, movement, behavior, and mood. From 2013 until his death in 2019, I was given drastically conflicting information about his prognosis based on the specialist (neurologist versus primary care physician versus hospital intensivist versus geriatrician) with whom I spoke. I learned quickly that I, as his caregiver, was often responsible for opening and guiding conversations about what to expect in terms of life span, quality of life, and potential benefits of treatment, as well as addressing and resolving the conflicting information we received. Opening these conversations—which are so necessary to plan for the present moment and the future—was an extraordinary source of anxiety for me, just as it was for countless caregivers who came to see me in the clinic. In fact, I found myself very frequently engaging in role-play exercises with caregivers in the clinic to allow them to practice having discussions about advance care planning with loved ones and healthcare providers (such as discussing a patient's goals of care and the type of treatment they might want to receive in the future), sessions that gave me vicarious practice in the same skill-building exercises. Not once as my dad's caregiver was I ever given professional guidance in navigating these conversations, though I certainly wish that I had been. As a result, assisting caregivers to strengthen their capacity to engage in advance care planning discussions with patients and healthcare teams was privately earmarked as an important area for me to address in my future work.

I also realized early on that until my dad's eventual death, I would be tasked with sitting with incredible uncertainty. I remember working with a caregiver whose wife had just been diagnosed with throat cancer. He shared with me that in some ways, he would have preferred to be told that there was no chance for a cure as opposed to her undergoing an aggressive treatment that might give her a small chance of her cancer going into remission. In the former scenario, he would know exactly what was going to happen, instead of navigating the ups and downs of recovery and subsequent cancer recurrence and what turned out to be several years of uncertainty before her death. I felt my stomach rise into my throat the moment he said that as I imagined my own dad's death, though a part of me also agreed with the sentiment. Sitting with uncertainty was challenging and painful; I had been doing it for decades and, at thirty, still found it almost as difficult as it was when I was ten, when I first started chewing on the idea of his death. While I knew that I could imagine my life after he was gone, I struggled to imagine surviving the intervening experiences.

One of the first caregivers in the clinic described his journey as one through liminal space. He and his partner had discussed the existential distress they were uniquely facing in their respective patient and caregiver roles, and they landed on the idea of the liminal space as encompassing both perspectives. The word *liminal* comes from the Latin word "limen," meaning threshold, or any point or place of entering or beginning. A liminal space is the time between *what was* and *what's next*. It is a place of transition, a season of waiting, and not knowing.

The caregiving journey *is* one through liminal space.

The caregiver is aware that (in many cases) the future decline or death of their loved one may eventually be unavoidable. They live in multiple realities: in one, trying to make the most of the present moment, addressing issues as they arise to promote the quality of life of the patient for whom they provide care; and in another, they anticipate a future without that loved one. Navigating this space, sitting with such uncertainty, is a key challenge for all caregivers and has subsequently been a driving force behind much of my research. This work endeavors to give caregivers the skills needed to navigate this liminal space and even use uncertainty as an opportunity to develop new strengths, from courageous communication practices to mindful self-compassion. For sure, in a heartbeat I would trade in my caregiving journey for just one more hug with my dad. But like so many caregivers, I have emerged from years of living with intense uncertainty as a much stronger, more confident, grounded, and peaceful version of myself.

Despite the profound complexity of living in this liminal space, within it exists the possibility to experience both meaning and suffering. At any one time, a caregiver may feel sadness, fear, hopelessness, anger, resentment, or anxiety, and intense love for the patient, pride in oneself, strength, gratitude, and hope. The positive and negative emotions are not mutually exclusive. The many extraordinary challenges of caregiving can coexist with connection to positive emotions, a sense of meaning and purpose, and the development of personal strengths. My dad and I had the most open, honest, and real connection. We left no stone unturned, no topic unaddressed, including this book. I was incredibly privileged in caring for my dad, privileged that the family member in need of my assistance was the one with whom I had the most extraordinary relationship. Caring for him afforded us the opportunity to learn more about each other, to continue to grow in our love and respect for one another until he took his last breath. It was the most exquisitely beautiful *and* painful experience of my life. As a result, much of the work I do is aimed at helping caregivers to connect to a sense of meaning and purpose in caregiving, and to recognize the potential benefits that can be derived from this role, whether they are the development of personal strengths or an improved relationship with their care partner. It's not about turning lemons to lemonade or the power of positive thinking. And it's not a process that requires you to have a relationship with your care partner like the one I had with my dad. Instead, it's about recognizing that in situations where we experience intense feelings of powerlessness, we can choose to connect to the meaning and purpose that is there, albeit often hidden at first. Now that my caregiving partnership with my dad has ended, the importance of assisting caregivers to cultivate this capacity is clearer to me than ever.

In 2013, when the intensity of what would be my personal caregiving journey became evident, I began sending emails to myself while standing by my dad's side during his hospital stays. Sometimes they contained thoughts that came to mind that paralleled the work I was doing professionally. Often, these were thoughts that I needed to express after difficult interactions with yet another fleeting medical team that I knew would land more safely and productively in my personal inbox than in a chart that would potentially label me as a difficult family member. Frequently these emails made me laugh as they documented the absurdity of many of the circumstances in which I found myself, such as the time I spent my morning in my dad's hospital bed trying to restrain him while he was having a seizure so the medical team could administer medications, all the while checking my phone to be sure a research grant application had been successfully submitted. Other times they included prayers to the universe to help me in a world of unknowns and endless medical outcomes that left me feeling powerless. I had a deep inner knowing when I began sending myself these emails back in 2013 that my personal experiences would profoundly shape my future work, though

I was not sure at the time exactly how. However, I felt confident that it was no accident that my personal and professional worlds seemed to be melding together in a spirited tango that would, after the final embrace, leave me deeply transformed.

Undeniably, the knowledge I gained while serving as "Allison," my dad's caregiver, and providing care as "Dr. Applebaum," has profoundly shaped me personally and professionally. Those emails I started sending myself in 2013 subsequently became the basis for much of what is written in the following pages. I knew before my dad's death that there was an important story to tell, about our caregiving journey as partners in his care, and more broadly of the master class in caregiving I had just experienced. The enormous responsibilities placed upon caregivers were well documented long before my caregiving journey began, though they were thoroughly brought to life for me by my lived experiences. I knew that I came to the role with many gifts, including a higher education, professional experience in healthcare, a supportive employer, and deeply caring friends, gifts that would mitigate some of the distress I was experiencing. Nonetheless, my caregiving responsibilities profoundly impacted every area of my life, from my relationships and financial security to my own physical and mental health. I experienced firsthand many of the themes I discuss in this book, including caregiver distress and burden, unmet needs, unpreparedness, invisibility, powerlessness, uncertainty, and financial toxicity. I saw myself as a microcosm of much larger issues faced by our nation, and recognized quickly that these challenges represented a national healthcare crisis. After my dad's death in 2019, I knew that this book would need to be written, both to help me grieve the loss of his life and make meaning of our journey as partners in care, and to shine a spotlight on the 53 million American caregivers who are essential to the functioning of our healthcare system and nation.

Stand By Me is a compilation of my dual experiences as a caregiver and as a clinician-scientist focused on addressing the needs of caregivers. Each of the following chapters weaves in narratives from my personal caregiving journey and over a decade of clinical experiences with caregivers, with reflections on the current research on caregiving science. If this journey is underway for you, my hope is that this book provides you with validation and guidance; if yours has not yet begun, my hope is that this book will prepare you to take on the caregiving role with courage. And if, like me, your caregiving responsibilities have ended, my hope is that this book helps you to connect—or reconnect—to the meaning and purpose that is available to us through caregiving.

CHAPTER 1

Becoming a Storyteller

Passing Strangers

Artist: Sarah Vaughan and Billy Eckstine
Written by Stanley Applebaum and Mel Mitchell, 1957

Caregivers are an essential extension of the healthcare team.

These words are too often implied between the lines of books on caregiving but are rarely stated directly. My responsibilities, like most caregivers, were vast. My presence too often meant the difference between life and death for my dad, and it *always* meant a difference in quality of life for my dad.

There is one element of this role and these responsibilities that is often overlooked, however. An element that is truly at the heart of what it means to be a caregiver. That is the responsibility to convey the patient's personhood to members of the healthcare team. To vividly illustrate who your care partner is, and what matters to them. Sharing their story and maintaining their legacy is central to your role, but rarely recognized formally. As you literally and metaphorically stand by your loved one, you are tasked with honoring the dignity of that patient, the dignity of the life that has been lived thus far, and the dignity of the life that can be lived in the future, through telling or helping to tell that patient's story. By doing so, you can help secure the most appropriate patient- and family-centered care that honors your loved one's values and goals.

You, then, are the keeper of a legacy.

❋ ❋ ❋

My storytelling would often start with the paramedics, who came in pairs to my dad's apartment within minutes of my calling 911. I would quickly share the events that precipitated that phone call, give my CliffsNotes version of his medical history, including his standing medications and most recent vital signs. They'd often ask if I was a physician given my manner of presenting my dad's case. I'd share that I wasn't, but instead through caregiving I had become seasoned in telling his story. I knew each time they arrived that I had to quickly convey the entire picture of my dad's health history and how his current state was a shift from baseline, and to emphasize the benefits of their taking us to the hospital where he received the majority of his outpatient care. But I often found myself using a few precious seconds to comment on a poster that hung near my dad's bed that included a picture of him and the subtitle, "*Stan Applebaum, the master of arranging, tells his secrets.*" I would mention my dad's joie de vivre, his creativity, and his desire to keep learning. During the ambulance ride to the hospital, I'd share more about what made my dad uniquely himself, such as his capacity to make everyone feel comfortable enough to share their dreams and disclose their deepest secrets, and to feel emotionally held and fully seen by him in the process. I wanted the paramedics to know that the body they were working on and transporting was not just a body but the home of an amazing person with an amazing story that was not ready to end.

This push inside me to tell his entire story would intensify once we arrived at the emergency room, first with the triage nurse who would speak with the paramedics and assign my dad to an area of the ER, and then with the nurse assigned to his case, a person I knew would likely become our close ally during the ER visit. As the nurse would draw blood and take urine samples to run cultures for infections, I would repeat what I shared with the paramedics. And then again, a third and fourth time, with the medical intern or resident who inevitably came next to the bed, and finally, with the attending physician who would direct my dad's medical care. With each subsequent telling of my dad's history, I found myself adding in more details about the medical picture and simultaneously striving to efficiently convey to the medical team who my dad was as a person, outside of his medical history. I realized during the first or second of what was eventually twenty-something ER visits that without me by his side, when my dad was disoriented or too ill to communicate on his own behalf, there was no way for any of these providers to truly *know* him, to know anything more than what they could physically see of him or read in his medical record. I knew that in those moments, without my conveying to the healthcare team who my dad was in terms of his personality and his drive for life, he could be labeled as another ninety-something-year-old man with multiple comorbidities and a likely poor prognosis. This label could significantly shape the care he would receive and the trajectory for his life. Without an advocate by his side in those vulnerable moments, he was at risk for being a passing stranger to the medical team.

The Importance of Holistic Care

The field of psycho-oncology in which I work, which unites psychiatry with oncology, was founded by Dr. Jimmie Holland. Dr. Holland was a true pioneer, a trailblazer, a brilliant educator and role model, psychiatrist, therapist, mentor, and colleague. She began the field of psycho-oncology in the late 1970s, created the first department of psychiatry housed in any cancer center (at Memorial Sloan Kettering Cancer Center), founded the American Psychosocial Oncology Society, cofounded the International Psycho-Oncology Society, and pressed for distress to be recognized as the sixth vital sign in medicine. Dr. Holland encouraged us all to recognize that, in order to comprehensively care for patients, we must attend to the emotional and psychological needs of those patients and of those who love and take care of them. She believed that understanding the experience of the human with cancer was just as important as understanding the biology of the cancer itself.

When I joined the faculty at Memorial Sloan Kettering, I had the good fortune of being placed in an office a few doors down from Dr. Holland, who up until her last days before her death in 2017 was working full-time and seeing patients late into the evening. One of the silver linings of my late-in-the day clinic schedule was my regular chats with Dr. Holland, which often began with her inviting me into her office and my commenting on the fresh flowers on her desk, which she picked regularly from her garden. In addition to being a botanist, Dr. Holland was also a wife, mother, grandmother, and baker, and in my opinion, a fashionista; she was, hands down, the best dressed of any faculty member at the hospital. Before asking about anything patient-related, Dr. Holland would make a point of looking me in the eyes and saying, "Now, how are you doing this evening?" It was a powerful open-ended question that, when asked by such a genuinely caring role model, allowed for an immense amount of self-disclosure. What stands out to me right now is her response when I shared the challenges I was facing in taking care of my dad, the challenges of his neurodegenerative disease, and feeling like it was a never-ending upward battle to secure comprehensive care for him, especially when he couldn't advocate for himself. She shared with me one of her favorite quotes, from Dr. Francis Peabody:

The secret of the care of the patient is in caring for the patient.[1]

She said what I needed to do, as my dad's caregiver, was make sure that everyone who was taking care of him knew who he was, so that they could *care* about who he was.

What Dr. Holland advocated for throughout her career, through the establishment of our field, and what she was emphasizing to me that evening, was holistic care. Holistic care involves treating a patient as a "whole" person instead of focusing on an illness or diagnosis, and considers psychological, cultural, and spiritual aspects when developing treatment plans. Holistic care is what Dr. Atul Gawande describes in *Being Mortal*, in which he argues that "The battle of being mortal is the battle to maintain the integrity of one's life.... Sickness and old age make the struggle hard enough. The professionals and institutions we turn to should not make it worse."[2] For such holistic care to be delivered, the provider needs to *know* the patient.

Holistic care is the type of care I was advocating for each time I spoke with the paramedics, the nurses, the medical interns, residents, and attending physicians. It is what I was advocating for each time I found myself showing time-stamped pictures and videos from the days leading up to ER visits, such as my dad discussing articles from the Tuesday *Science Times* he had recently read, to assist my narrative. I wanted his providers to *meet* Stan Applebaum. Inevitably, the staff who got to know my dad responded to him and me in a way that demonstrated a different tenor of care, and that translated into what felt like more personalized medical care, and certainly more responsiveness and greater communication with me.

*   *   *

My dad, Stanley Seymour Applebaum, was born on March 1, 1922. He began studying the piano at age seven after he fell out of a tree and broke his pinkie finger. His doctor suggested that tapping the player piano my grandparents had at home might be a good form of physical therapy. Little did that doctor know that his prescription would lead to the beginning of a musical career that would span three-quarters of a century and touch millions of lives. In addition to his talent as a pianist, my dad had a special gift for orchestration (the art of arranging a musical composition for performance by an orchestra or other ensemble) and arranging (the adaptation of an existing composition for performance on an instrument, voice, or combination of instruments for which it was not originally composed), which led to his writing hundreds of orchestrations and arrangements for great artists including Ben E. King, Neil Sedaka, Connie Francis, Della Reese, Sarah Vaughn, Brook Benton, Joanie Sommers, and Bobby Vinton. Perhaps most notable are his arrangements for Ben E. King's "Stand By Me" and "Spanish Harlem," The Drifters' "Save the Last Dance for Me" and "This Magic Moment," Brian Hyland's "Sealed with a Kiss," and Neil Sedaka's "Breaking Up Is Hard to Do," "Stairway to Heaven," and "Calendar Girl." The unforgettable string interlude in the middle of "Stand By Me" that sounds like a full orchestra was my dad's composition, something he wrote on a whim one night while playing around with how rich and full he could make just several stringed instruments sound while played in unison. Little did he know it was a string line that would be beloved by generations to come.

In addition to creating orchestrations for the United States Army when he served in World War II, and after for the Navy and the Air Force, my dad wrote music for Radio City Music Hall, Broadway, NBC, CBS, and the New York and London Philharmonics. He was also a prolific writer of over 1,500 commercials, most notably the jingle "Pan Am Makes the Going Great," for which he won a Clio Award in 1968 and upon which George Balanchine choreographed the ballet *PAMTGG* for the New York City Ballet. In the later and "quieter" phase of his career, as he described it, my dad became the principal arranger and orchestrator for the New York Pops, the orchestra housed at Carnegie Hall in New York City. Pretty much every show played by the Pops from the early nineties until 2005 was infused with a touch of Stan Applebaum.

The magnitude of my father's musical career is underscored (pun intended) by what the New York Public Library for the Performing Arts would say in 2018 after he donated his music and scores so that others could learn from his writing: The music took up twenty-seven linear feet of space in the Special Collections Archive. That is a *lot* of music. As if all this musical creativity was not enough, my dad also authored a series of children's books in the 1970s focused on science and nature. And in the last ten years of his life, including those he spent confined to a hospital bed, he wrote over five hundred poems and children's stories. He never stopped writing. He never stopped creating.

There's a part of my dad's story, however, that's not mentioned in his many credits, biographical pieces, interviews, oral histories, or Wikipedia pages. It's another part of his story that I wanted to convey to the medical teams, though perhaps it was conveyed silently by the fact that whenever possible, our hands were tightly intertwined. My dad was a prolific, creative, and masterful musician. But more important than that to me, he was an extraordinarily talented father.

When I came into the picture on a cold evening in November of 1981, my dad was nearly sixty. He had already had an incredibly successful career, and much of his fame had been achieved years before. Perhaps in part due to his age, his accomplishments, and his experiences during his first sixty years, I was blessed with the gift of my dad investing much of his creative energy into parenting me and my older brother. He loved being a dad; he loved teaching us how to play the piano, how to read, how to ride a bike, how to fish, how to cook, how to do home repairs. He was curious, always asking questions like, "How does that bird fly?" or "What kinds of clouds are those?" We talked about science, art, history. We talked about music, his career, and the ups and downs of his life. We talked about everything. My dad was fully, one hundred percent, completely my best friend, my closest confidant, my teacher, my mentor, my sounding board, my shoulder to lean on. There was no topic we couldn't touch on, nothing too sensitive. He modeled for me openness, vulnerability, and what it means to be human: not perfect, flawed and beautiful.

I was ten years old when I realized that my dad was older. I'll never forget that day, because it's a day that changed my life, or my inner world, dramatically. I was standing outside the Plaza Hotel in New York with my dad and my brother, and for some reason the topic of my dad's age came up. He was, at the time, seventy. I remember being initially confused when I equated my dad's age with being old; he was the opposite of old in my eyes. He was active and working full-time and driving and doing everything that dads do. And he had an almost full head of hair. That day, however, changed my vision and how I saw the world; from then until he died, there wasn't a day when the possibility of my dad's death didn't cross my mind in some way. During my adolescence and teenage years that awareness would translate into a variety of thoughts, like when I watched him go into the kitchen to get a late-night snack of Häagen-Dazs ice cream and thought "that's the bite that's going to lead to the heart attack." Many of my thoughts were irrational. But many, not. He was a source of balance in what was an occasionally chaotic adolescence. He seemed to be my compass, my GPS; I felt like I had enough oxygen to breathe deeply when I was around him, and I was terrified of losing that supply.

Like so many partners in care, I began thinking about my dad's health—and death—long before I became his caregiver. However, these thoughts and fears became much more rational as I entered adulthood and he entered what was unequivocally "old age," despite his continuing to work and drive and be active and fully self-sufficient into his nineties. He was living on what my maternal grandmother would call borrowed time. He and I both knew that. And yet, he was still here, living life as fully as possible.

*   *   *

Twenty-four years after I stood outside the Plaza with my dad and brother and internalized an association between my dad's age and death, those early-childhood cognitions were replaced by concerns about how I could ensure that my dad received the type of care advocated for by Dr. Holland. By that time, I had already become seasoned at telling his story, having had practice during the approximately fifteen trips to the hospital we had already taken as partners in care.

It was a Sunday morning, and I had just arrived at my then ninety-four-year-old dad's apartment with a cranberry muffin and decaf coffee in hand, a treat we had shared since the days of his driving me to ballet class decades earlier. I arrived to find him doing Pilates exercises in bed using my TheraBand, and he was counting his leg lifts in Tagalog, the native language of the home health aides I had hired to assist us since my mom's death. When he had finished exercising, I sat next to him and we proceeded to collaboratively complete the *New York Times* crossword puzzle, albeit slowly, while listening to WQXR, the classical music radio station that served as the backdrop to our then thirty-four-year-long relationship. Interspersed with discussing clues to the puzzle was commentary about the composer we had just heard, often about how that composer influenced a piece my dad had written.

Twenty-four hours later, bacteria crawled their way into the opening of my dad's suprapubic catheter (a tube that was inserted into his bladder to assist with urination), and when I arrived at his bedside, he was difficult to rouse. This, we found out later, was because he was becoming septic; that is, a bacterial infection had moved from his bladder straight into his bloodstream and he was losing blood pressure and adequate oxygenation of his brain. I called an ambulance and soon after found myself in the ER where I once again was tasked with serving as his eyes, ears, and mouth, and helping the medical team to understand what a significant shift from baseline my dad's current state was. The medical resident who initially examined him looked at me with skepticism as I described the events of the prior day. The man lying in the stretcher was unable to keep his eyes open or speak in that moment. He did not resemble the man who was committed to living each day to its fullest, to continuing to learn and grow, despite his limitations.

When a patient is brought to the hospital and is unable to advocate for themself, assumptions can be made about that patient's capacity for meaningful life and what meaningful life can look like for that patient. Age and cognitive status are two key drivers of these assumptions that caregivers must combat, assumptions often based on incomplete data that healthcare professionals are vulnerable to in fast-paced environments. As my dad's caregiver, I quickly learned how critical it was for me to help the medical team to know my dad, to personalize the body lying on the stretcher in front of them, to help them understand what a significant shift his current state was from his day-to-day functioning, and to appreciate the vast goals my dad had for the remainder of his life. I knew that, in those moments when he was unable to advocate for himself, I was responsible for telling his story, and making it matter to those taking care of him.

Had I not been there to share my dad's story, it would have been impossible for that resident and anyone else involved in my dad's care to not rely—at least partially—on assumptions about what care was appropriate to deliver. It would also have been nearly impossible for members of the healthcare team to collect the information that would eventually land in the History of Present Illness (HPI) section of his medical record. The HPI section is an area that you, as the caregiver, are often responsible for filling in. This is the section where most of the information that you share about your care partner's story, including their medical history, current and past diagnoses, medications, and especially the events leading up to the ER visit, will land. These, and other key pieces of information you should have whenever you bring a loved one to the ER, are outlined below.

"Must Know" Information for Caregivers for ER Visits

- Patient's date of birth and Social Security number
- Patient's self-identified gender if different than that assigned at birth
- Patient's current and past medical and psychiatric diagnoses
- Patient's current—and recent changes in—medications (including psychiatric medications) and dosing instructions

- Patient's symptoms and how long they have been experiencing them, including recent changes in vital signs (blood pressure, pulse, respiratory rate, and temperature)
- Patient's current use of other substances (e.g., alcohol, marijuana)
- Patient's allergies (e.g., to latex, medications, foods)
- Patient's recent surgeries or other medical procedures
- Patient's cognitive/mobility status at baseline and current cognitive/mobility status
- Patient's communication capacity and any factors that hinder communication (e.g., hearing loss)
- History of falls
- If the patient has a healthcare proxy and you are not that person, the contact information for that person
- Whether or not the patient has signed a Do-Not-Resuscitate (DNR) or Do-Not-Intubate (DNI) order, has any other advance directives executed (e.g., living will), and the patient's preferences, values, or goals of care that would be essential for staff to know (e.g., does not want blood transfusions)
- Name and contact information for the patient's outpatient providers such as primary care physicians and specialists like cardiologists and urologists
- Patient's health insurance information

For my dad's HPI, this meant sharing his current diagnosis of Lewy body disease as well as mild heart and kidney failure (both of which made him more acutely sensitive to the onset of sepsis); his list of five standing medications with dosing (timing and amount) instructions; the fact that I had come home to find him difficult to rouse and documented upward shifts in his vital signs (blood pressure, pulse, temperature) that likely indicated some sort of infection taking hold; and perhaps most importantly, what his functioning was like just a day before, and the fact that my father was not DNR (that is, he had not signed a Do-Not-Resuscitate order). In sharing these details, I was able to meaningfully convey what my dad's quality of life looked like just a day earlier, and how important it was for him to be able to achieve more life like that. Had I not continued to stand by his side after the IV antibiotics kicked in, it would have been nearly impossible for my dad—given his natural age- and illness-related hearing and vision loss—to communicate effectively in a busy emergency room. In that moment it was clear to me that, in addition to all my other various responsibilities, being my dad's caregiver meant honoring his wishes and advocating for him through tirelessly conveying who my dad was and what made him uniquely him.

This was a profound responsibility, as it may be for you. The weight of it often felt heavy on my shoulders but at the same time, it inspired and motivated me to continue to stand by his side in my moments of greatest physical and emotional exhaustion.

In *The Soul of Care*, Dr. Arthur Kleinman speaks of a moral problem that results from the inattention of healthcare professionals to the stories behind patients and illness. This moral problem arises in part from the disparity in the experience of the family caregiver, who has intimate knowledge of the patient's personhood, and that of healthcare providers, who, he writes, "enter that experience only for brief, fragmented clinical moments, usually without context or meaning, unless they stop long enough to ask, and listen."[3]

Many factors contribute to these fragmented clinical moments, and most are not because healthcare professionals are disinterested in their patients. Instead, they result from limitations of the broader systems within which such healthcare providers work. For example, time urgency describes most triage processes in ERs, and staff often must collect an immense amount of clinical data quickly, which traditionally precludes learning more than the basic medical picture of the patient in front of them. Second, most ER staff are wearing multiple hats, covering many patients at a time and multitasking to ensure the greatest number of patients are seen and ideally triaged out. Third, clinical productivity expectations for clinicians are ever increasing. Combined, these factors limit the amount of time each provider can spend with each patient. If there has been a poor hand-off from community providers, ER staff are starting from scratch in learning about the patients in front of them, further intensifying the need to quickly gather clinical data and precluding the opportunity to use some of that time to learn more about patients' personhood. Indeed, my own experience working as a clinical psychology intern staffing a psychiatric emergency room was predominantly spent contacting primary care physicians and outside mental health providers to try to collect information about patients who arrived without caregivers.

It is for these reasons that your presence is particularly crucial in a busy ER. Looking back, time urgency, periodic understaffing, poor handoff from outside providers, and healthcare staff burnout all contributed to situations in which my dad was at risk for being a passing stranger to his ER team. In effect, it often became my job to compensate for the overcrowding and understaffing of the ER. I would spend hours standing by his stretcher, fearful to leave to use the bathroom or get food. I knew that if I were to miss a rounding team's visit it might delay my dad's care by days. And I wasn't alone. Inevitably throughout the ER were many worn-out caregivers, anxiously standing by their loved ones' stretchers, sending knowing glances to one another. They were striving to do exactly what I was doing. Back then I had the thought that we should be given a badge or a sticker, something that would identify us as the caregiver, the linchpin of that patient's care. Instead, we often felt invisible and undervalued, feelings that amplified our already high levels of distress.

As I did, you can serve as the missing link in communication and information flow between multiple teams and on behalf of your care partner, especially if they are unable to advocate for themselves. Though repeatedly telling your care partner's story may become frustrating at times, you will likely realize that you are playing a key role in helping them to secure the care they need through helping their providers get to know them. The more efficiently you can achieve this, the faster your care partner can receive care that is responsive to their needs and sensitive to their goals.

As you share their story, I encourage you to draw on one of the most powerful tools for caregivers, one that was particularly important for me when my dad was unable to advocate for himself: *the time-stamped video*. I would take out my phone and show, for example, a video from three days earlier of my dad walking up and down the hallway outside our apartment, or him sitting at the piano the prior week, or him walking down the boardwalk by the New Jersey shore with minimal assistance a year after he was in a coma and I was told by many physicians to not expect to speak with him ever again. It was in these moments that I found myself striving to continue to share my dad's story, to help the medical professional in front of me appreciate what a shift from baseline my dad's current functioning was, and to give context for his stated goals of care, those I was conveying on his behalf.

When providers can connect with patients, either directly with that patient or through a caregiver, the care becomes personalized, more intimate. Healthcare providers can then do exactly what Dr. Holland suggested; they can more deeply and authentically *care*. Then, the emotional experience for all involved can change, and the emotional distance between the healthcare professional and patient can be shortened. I witnessed this repeatedly, especially when my dad was disoriented and unable to communicate but when members of his care team took the time to get to know him through me. Those providers—from the aides who changed the dirty linens, to the lab techs who took his blood, to the residents and attendings who developed a medical care plan—not only seemed to provide care more empathically but appeared to emotionally soften in the process. Allowing healthcare professionals to know my dad connected them with the human in the stretcher and I hope, to the unique emotional gifts that are possible through patient care.

Certainly, my job of telling my dad's story and engaging members of the healthcare team in this story was aided by the uniqueness of his musical legacy. But it was never the celebrity nature of his story that mattered most in my sharing. Instead, it was his drive for life, humor, childlike curiosity, exuberance, and desire to make the most of every moment presented to him that I wanted others to connect to. And these are the unique facets of your loved ones' personalities, what makes them uniquely them, that will be important for you to share as a caregiver. Indeed, it was less about what my dad *did* and more about who he *was* in the world, what it was like to *be* Stan Applebaum that was most impactful for me to share.

My life has been divided into two eras, and there are only a small number of family and friends who truly got to know Stanley Applebaum, my dad, instead of Stan Applebaum, the world-famous composer, arranger, and orchestrator. I want his legacy to be kept alive, to reverberate past his string lines and into everyone's hearts. So, while I am writing this book to support and advocate for caregivers, each word on these pages is written dually to ensure that my dad's story is not forgotten and will continue for generations to come.

CHAPTER 2

Embracing the Change

Goodbye Summer

Artist: Joanie Sommers
Produced and Arranged by Stan Applebaum, 1963

For some of you, stepping into the caregiving role may happen incrementally. Perhaps it will begin with your offering time-limited assistance with specific health-related tasks that eventually turns into a dynamic with a care partner relying completely on you for care. For others of you, a specific event may occur that will completely redirect your life orbit to one that centers around taking care of someone else. Or maybe you cannot pinpoint the moment you became a caregiver, but you know that caregiving has become a defining feature of your life.

In the winter of 2011, I received a phone call that I had begun to dread a few years prior. It was a Saturday morning and my dad had taken a drive down to our family house by the New Jersey shore, as he had done for years on Saturday mornings. He usually arrived at the house by ten in the morning and would call me shortly after getting settled. Around ten thirty I hadn't heard from him and started to worry, imagining the worst, and soon after received a call from an unknown number with a New Jersey area code. I didn't have to answer to know it was bad. As soon as I said hello my body froze; the voice on the other end said, "Ma'am, this is Lieutenant Scott from the New Jersey State Police. There's been an accident." I wish he had started with what he eventually would tell me: "Your father is okay; remarkably, he's not severely injured." My dad's car was hit on the passenger side after it had drifted into another lane, and that entire side of the car had been destroyed. He was saved by his airbag and perhaps some other higher intervention, I imagine, because judging by a picture of the wrecked car a few days later, he should not have walked away from the scene. The officer told me my dad was scared and disoriented but was able to give the police my number.

I don't exactly remember making a conscious decision to become my dad's caregiver, to take responsibility for all aspects of his medical care, his well-being, and eventually his survival. However, when I reflect on the events of the decade starting in 2009 with my return to New York City after graduate school until his death in 2019, this accident stands out as the defining moment: that day, when he gave the police my phone number, my dad chose to make me responsible for his well-being.

Who Are Caregivers?

According to the National Alliance for Caregiving, caregivers of adults are defined as those who provide unpaid care, as described by the following question:

> At any time in the last 12 months, has anyone in your household provided *unpaid care to a relative or friend 18 years or older to help them take care of themselves?* This may include

helping with personal needs or household chores. It might be managing a person's finances, arranging for outside services, or visiting regularly to see how they are doing. This adult need not live with you.[1]

My guess is that for many of you, your answer to this question is yes. If so, you're in good company: As of 2020, at least 53 million Americans identify as caregivers, and nearly one-quarter of caregivers provide care to two or more people. And these numbers don't include the additional 3.4 million caregivers who are children and adolescents in the United States today.

As caregivers, most of you are providing care to blood relatives, like parents or children, though many of you are taking care of spouses and partners and members of your chosen family. Nearly half of you provide care to someone seventy-five years of age or older, and nearly two-thirds of you are taking care of individuals with long-term physical conditions, such as the neurodegenerative disease my dad had. You're also likely to be taking care of someone with multiple conditions.

What Do Caregivers Do?

Whenever I lecture on caregiving, I show a slide with the question, "What Do Caregivers Do?" The answer I share is *everything*. According to the National Alliance for Caregiving, caregivers provide care for an average of four and a half years, though for almost one-third, the role is one that lasts for more than five years, and up to ten years or more for many.[2] As they are for so many, these were extraordinarily intense years for me. Exhausting years. Life- and soul-changing years. During this time, caregivers spend nearly twenty-five hours a week on average providing care, though one-quarter provide forty-one or more hours of care a week, which means this is undoubtedly a full-time job often conducted in addition to full-time paid employment. At times, this certainly was the case for me.

Frequently, caregivers will tell me that they don't necessarily identify as caregivers. Instead, they'll say, "I'm just doing what any [partner or son or daughter or sibling or parent or friend] would do." But then I ask about the different types of help they give to their care partners, and inevitably I hear about the following categories of very clear caregiving tasks:

Activities of Daily Living (ADLs) are basic self-care tasks, such as helping your loved one to get dressed, bathed, or out of bed and into a wheelchair. About two-thirds of caregivers help with ADLs, and many of these responsibilities can be physically taxing and require training to be completed without injury. One of the ADLs caregivers of adult patients find particularly physically and emotionally challenging is assisting with toileting and changing diapers. If this type of task is on your to-do list, I hope to help normalize some of the feelings that might be coming up for you about it, like resentment and disgust.

Instrumental Activities of Daily Living (IADLs) are activities that allow an individual to live independently in the community, such as shopping, housework, and managing finances. Nearly all caregivers assist with IADLs. While perhaps on their own these are not necessarily the most stressful to do, they can become burdensome when added on top of other responsibilities.

If you have a network assisting with care, IADLs are often the responsibilities that can be delegated. This was the case for me and my family. While my brother didn't take over day-to-day caregiving responsibilities after our mom died, he was able to help meaningfully with IADLs, including dropping off groceries, facilitating transportation to doctors' appointments, and contributing financially to help cover the cost of my dad's home health aides. Since support for IADLs may be more easily shared than other caregiving responsibilities, when offers of help come to you from family and friends, I not only want you to say yes immediately but I want you to specify which IADL they can assist with, such as setting up a meal train or managing home repairs. Crossing one or two of these tasks off your list can make a significant difference for you in terms of your energy and bandwidth for assisting with more hands-on caregiving.

Medical and Nursing Tasks deserve their own category as they are conducted by nearly two-thirds of caregivers and are the responsibilities for which many caregivers feel least prepared. These range from the simplest tasks, such as taking blood pressure or temperature readings using digital machines, to more complex activities like changing wound dressings and administering injectable medications. Most caregivers will, at some point, assist patients with medical or nursing tasks, and while these can be accomplished with training, such training is routinely absent.

Additionally, you will likely spend a significant amount of time and energy communicating with healthcare professionals and advocating for your care partner with a variety of providers and services. Looking back, there was rarely a day between 2014 and 2019 when I was not fielding phone calls from one of my dad's physicians, visiting nurses, or home health aides, or from Medicaid.

If you're like two-thirds of caregivers today, you are doing all the above while also trying to maintain paid employment. Sadly, I've lost count of the number of caregivers I've worked with who received a warning about performance or attendance at work because of accommodations taken due to caregiving. I was lucky that some of my work responsibilities could be accomplished outside the physical walls of Memorial Sloan Kettering. Had this not been the case, my caregiving journey would have been exponentially more difficult and like too many caregivers today, I would have been forced to make the impossible decision between paid employment and caregiving.

So, as a caregiver you're doing *a lot*. And my guess is you may feel like you don't necessarily have a choice in taking on these responsibilities. This certainly was how I felt the day I received the phone call from the New Jersey State Police, and how many of the caregivers I see in clinic feel. This is important, because feeling like you had a choice in taking on the caregiving role can dramatically shape your emotional experience of caregiving: According to the National Alliance for Caregiving, caregivers who report having no choice face more complex care situations and increased stress compared to caregivers who feel a sense of choice in this role.[3]

This sense of choice in caregiving also appears to diminish with time; nearly two-thirds of caregivers providing five or more years of care report feeling no choice in this role. Moreover, choice seems to be associated with employment; caregivers who work more than thirty hours a week report more often feeling like they have no choice in taking on caregiving than those who are unemployed or working fewer hours.[4] A significant burden clearly falls on caregivers who already shoulder significant responsibility. Choice in caregiving is also often culturally constructed, and in some cultures providing care for one's family is an expected and accepted part of the life cycle, allowing for less of a sense of choice.[5] And perhaps not surprisingly, given the traditionally gendered nature of caregiving, women report not having choice more frequently than men.[6]

While caregiving can at times be challenging for all, research also suggests that the experience is very much impacted by one's age and development. Caregivers are, on average, 49.4 years of age.[7] However, one-quarter are between ages 18 and 34, 23 percent are between ages 35 and 49, 35 percent are between ages 50 and 64, 12 percent are between ages 65 and 74, and 7 percent are over age 75. Dr. Kristin Litzelman, a population health scientist at the University of Wisconsin, has studied the unique experiences of caregivers across the life span.[8] She notes that early adulthood, broadly defined as ages eighteen to forty-four, is a time of self-discovery and developing independence in which individuals are exploring their identity and making choices related to marriage, family, education, and career. It's a period during which caregiving is particularly developmentally non-normative.[9] Not only can caregiving have a significant impact on young adults while they serve as caregivers but it can also adversely impact their lives moving forward.

Young adult caregivers are particularly vulnerable to life disruptions, and many report having to quit working, missing job promotion opportunities, and having long-term career goals being negatively impacted due to caregiving demands.[10] These career and employment choices in early adulthood have a ripple effect on later opportunities. At a time when their peers are establishing and advancing their careers, such employment changes may have a dramatic cumulative impact on career advancement potential, lifetime earning potential, or retirement savings.[11] According to Litzelman, caregiving may also be a strain on romantic relationships and family functioning, or act as a barrier to development in this area.[12] Caregivers often face time constraints and are challenged to make time for self-care or dating, and many young adult caregivers report difficulty establishing or maintaining dating relationships[13] and may give up on dating entirely.[14] Among those in committed relationships, some report that caregiving negatively impacted their relationship,[15] specifically indicating strains related to having less time for their significant other or their partner being unsupportive of their caregiving role.[16] Not surprisingly, the death of a parent is a challenge for many young adults[17] and may be particularly intense for those who provided care to parents before their deaths. This certainly was the case for me.

According to Litzelman, at middle age (forty-five to sixty-four), many working adults are reaching the apex of their careers, but caregivers in this age group often face complicated decisions regarding their working lives.[18] They are not yet eligible for many retirement benefits and their family may rely on their job for income or health insurance; at the same time, the responsibilities of caregiving may make it challenging to continue working full- or even part-time. Added to financial and employment challenges, caregivers in middle age may also experience the onset of their own health problems, as chronic diseases become more common in middle age[19] and can negatively impact their ability to carry out caregiving-related responsibilities. Too often I hear about new medical diagnoses or preexisting conditions, like high blood pressure or diabetes, worsening during an intense caregiving period for caregivers in this age group.

Caregiving is far more normative in older age than other life stages, and older caregivers tend to have a greater amount of caregiving-specific support and validation through common experiences among friends and acquaintances. Reductions in work and childcare responsibilities leave later-life caregivers with fewer competing demands and more time and financial resources for caregiving.[20] However, caregivers over age seventy-five may be particularly vulnerable to illness and physical decline that impact their capacity to take care of themselves, as well as a loved one with a chronic or life-limiting illness.[21]

The unique challenges caregivers experience across the life span underscore the benefits of support groups. If you are a young adult caregiver, support groups can help you to feel less alone and more "normal" despite the distinct changes and challenges you might be facing. You may realize through hearing the stories of other young adult caregivers how your caregiving journey and experiences have influenced your growth. You may find, for example, that despite your potentially getting "off track" with certain life goals such as building a romantic partnership, you have learned the deepest meaning of love and commitment through caregiving, and eventually this value will serve you well when you have the bandwidth to date. If you are a caregiver in middle age balancing multiple caregiving responsibilities, you may find that connecting with others who understand what it feels like to be pulled in a million directions can be validating. And if you are an older adult caregiver, support groups can help to bolster peer support that commonly diminishes as we age. Ultimately, while each of your caregiving journeys is unique, sharing your experience with others will help to highlight commonalities and promote connection, validation, and growth.

*   *   *

Jennifer came to see me in 2015. At the time of her first visit, she was thirty-one, single, and working in financial services. Her sixty-year-old mother, Maria, had been recently diagnosed with advanced melanoma, and while Maria lived at home on Long Island with Jennifer's father, Jennifer shared with me that it was almost expected, without question, that she would take on most caregiving responsibilities. Her parents were Chinese immigrants, and Jennifer remembered watching her mother take care of her grandmother when her grandmother was in the end stages of Alzheimer's disease, and the sense of honor and responsibility her mother expressed at the time.

But instead of honor, Jennifer felt a deep sense of resentment. She felt that she had no choice but to help. Her father, Mùchén, was sixty-five, and although he was a retired engineer, he had recently taken a part-time job teaching at a community college. He assumed that Jennifer would be able to step in so that he could continue to work. This meant that Jennifer needed to travel from Manhattan to Long Island multiple times a week to accompany Maria to appointments at a regional site for chemotherapy infusions, and eventually immunotherapy. These aggressive treatments left her mother weak and nauseous, and Jennifer quickly assumed responsibility for her parents' home as well, doing the grocery shopping, cooking, and cleaning. While initially she found respite through work and in being able to return to her apartment in the city, after several months of commuting, repeatedly traveling back into the city became too exhausting. She also began to worry about leaving her mother home alone during the days when she was feeling weak and sick from treatments. This, combined with Jennifer's increasing difficulty with focusing on work during the day due to fielding numerous calls from the hospital and checking in on her mother, led her to realize that she needed to take time off from work. She was initially able to do so by protecting her job through the Family Medical Leave Act (FMLA), but after several months the coverage ran out and Jennifer was forced to decide between returning to work full-time or leaving altogether. She shared with me that she was desperate to return to work and her old life; she wanted to earn money and spend time in the city dating and focusing on her future. But her sense of obligation to her parents—and the reality of no one else being available to serve as a caregiver—would make this almost impossible. Jennifer ultimately left work altogether, gave up her apartment, and moved in with her parents. This allowed her to be fully present with her mother, which turned out in some ways to be a gift as, eight months later, her mother's cancer stopped responding to treatments and she transitioned to hospice care.

The shift to full-time caregiving, however, had a profound impact on Jennifer. Helping her mother to bathe or use the toilet was emotionally and physically challenging, and she became increasingly resentful of her father for not helping more. Her social circle narrowed severely, and she put dating completely on hold. Without work and income, the debt from her student loans continued to grow, and she feared that it would be challenging to secure a similarly high-paying and growth-promoting job in the future with a gap on her résumé. Jennifer began having difficulty falling and staying asleep, and she spent much of her waking time worrying about the future. After her mother's death in home hospice, Jennifer felt "boxed in," required to remain at home on Long Island with her father. She struggled to balance her grief with her resentment of him, and her growing recognition that her own life goals had been severely sidetracked. She was completely burned out.

As it was for Jennifer during our work together, learning how to remain connected to valued activities and roles outside of caregiving—like spending even small amounts of time connecting with friends and exercising—is an essential tool for you to cope with increasing caregiving demands and feeling boxed in. This is particularly important when your existing roles shift due to caregiving. Similarly, identifying the strengths you bring to caregiving, such as strong communication skills or emotional intelligence, can help you cultivate confidence and even pride in your ability to carry forward this role. These strengths will, no doubt, serve you well in all areas of your life, not just caregiving.

The Impact of Caregiving on You

Like Jennifer, because of the vast responsibilities and intensity of caregiving, along with limited support, most caregivers experience what is often called *caregiver burden*. This term refers to all the ways in which the caregiving role can potentially negatively impact you.

Importantly, there is no International Classification of Diseases (ICD) code for caregiver burden; that is, it is not a billable health condition and it is not formally recognized as a health problem. However, every caregiver reading this knows that it certainly is one.

Burden has been described as the negative reaction to the impact of providing care on caregivers' social, occupational, and personal roles, as well as on their physical and emotional health.[22] Burden results from an imbalance between the objective and subjective demands of caregiving and your coping resources. It is experienced when the number of responsibilities on your plate far surpasses your internal and external resources. Each of you has certainly dealt with burden in some context before. I personally have yet to meet an adult who has led a burden-free life, and in many ways, we've normalized the experience of burden, especially as we take on the expected responsibilities of adulthood. However, when burden endures, when it intensifies, and when it's left unaddressed, it can have profound effects on you, including changes in your mental and physical health.

Psychological Burden

As a caregiver, you will likely experience some form of psychological distress,[23] and this distress can be more severe than the distress experienced by your care partner. This can include anxiety, such as intense worry and fear and physical symptoms like a racing heart, stomachaches, and muscle tension. Depression is also common and can involve feelings of sadness and hopelessness, a loss of interest or pleasure in activities that you once enjoyed, and difficulty sleeping. Psychological distress in caregivers can also include symptoms of post-traumatic stress disorder (PTSD), such as experiencing intrusive memories and images from earlier moments of caregiving, hypervigilance or being on "high alert" for something going wrong, and irritability. Like war veterans and other trauma survivors, as a caregiver, you are often exposed to a life threat—to your loved one. Repeatedly witnessing threats to your loved one's life puts you at risk for experiencing vicarious or secondhand trauma. In fact, many caregivers must manage living with these trauma symptoms while continuing to spend time in the environments—hospitals, doctors' offices, homes—in which the traumas occurred, or which are filled with reminders of the trauma.

A key contributor to psychological distress is isolation, and one of the most common themes I hear from caregivers is how isolated they feel. This certainly was the case for me, and perhaps this is something you have felt as well. You may have limited opportunities to socialize and find it too stressful to schedule social events on top of your caregiving responsibilities. For so many caregivers, the uncertainty of care partners' illnesses or treatments prevents them from being able to make social plans in advance. Moreover, caregivers frequently describe feeling misunderstood by even close friends and finding simple conversations invalidating. One caregiver powerfully depicted this experience of caregiving and isolation in the following way:

> I feel like I traveled to another planet and learned how to speak Martian, and I've been sent back to Earth and am expected to remember how to speak English. I'm expected to know how to function in this world. Conversations about the mundane, questions like "Where did you get that jacket?" or "What summer camp is your son going to?" seem so trivial when my recent history is plagued by harrowing memories of [my daughter] lying in a stretcher in the hospital hooked up to machines.

Well-meaning friends and acquaintances may say things that are trite or unintentionally offensive, making it less and less emotionally safe and welcoming for you to socialize in the first place. All these factors may lead you to avoid socializing altogether, further contributing to your isolation.

I remember a moment that punctuated my feelings of isolation and the rift I perceived between my experience and that of my peers. It was December 2017, and I had come home early from work on a Thursday after the home health aide texted me a picture of my dad's catheter bag filled with blood and news that his temperature was rising quickly. It was clear there was a UTI spreading, and if we did not get him to the hospital, he would be at risk for becoming septic. So, I called 911, and a half hour later as we rode in the ambulance across town, we got stuck in traffic. I was told sirens would only be used if my dad's condition deteriorated en route to the ER. A minute into the traffic jam—on the long list of excruciatingly long minutes in my life—the siren went off, and I was left feeling shaky and breathless. I tried to hide my tears by looking out the window, and there on the street just ten feet away from the ambulance was a group of my colleagues heading to our department's holiday party. I so longed to be with them, to enjoy the fun and connectedness that these gatherings can bring and to feel free to just be present with peers. I was sad and angry and frustrated all at once. I felt completely left out, completely isolated. No one in that moment could join me in how I was feeling, and the one person who had consistently provided emotional mirroring was fading in the stretcher in front of me. How ridiculous, I thought to myself, to focus on my feelings of isolation when the echoing sirens conveyed the possibility of my dad's life ending in that ambulance. The reality of my dad's health forced me back to the present moment, but deep down the lump inside remained.

What I did in that moment—my pushing down my varied emotional needs—can also contribute to burden. Inevitably, you will have many moments when your emotional needs must take a back seat to the events unfolding in front of you. This is real. And this is why I find the oft-repeated oxygen mask metaphor occasionally invalidating—you know, the idea that you *must* put on your oxygen mask before you can take care of others? In moments of crisis, or even moments when you're juggling a million caregiving and non-caregiving responsibilities, it's almost always impossible to put on an oxygen mask. However, once there is a calm moment, a chance to breathe, taking time to replenish your oxygen is a good idea. And that includes allowing the expression of all the emotions that have been pushed down, avoided, and neglected. Taking space to express these emotions will help to prevent mental health challenges down the line. Looking back, I know that if it weren't for my allowing myself to express my emotions—frequently with my friends, my dad, and my therapist—I would have certainly experienced a significant worsening of my mental health and likely, my ability to take care of my dad.

In addition to isolation, psychological burden for many caregivers is driven by a loss of control over one's life. One caregiver who was taking care of her husband shared powerfully:

I can't help but feel like my envisioned trajectory of where I'd thought I'd be in my career right now has been completely derailed. I feel like each month that passes by is another dream deferred.

My own experience of burden was certainly driven largely by the loss of control over my own life, the growing feeling that I was being stripped of my own life and goals. I longed not only to go to holiday parties but to be able to go to work and simply focus on work projects for an entire day. I longed to be able to make plans for a vacation in the future but knew there was a significant likelihood these plans would fall through. I longed to be "normal." My caregiver role took that away from me. During my dad's long ER visits, I would often scroll through social media on my phone and feel like I was a fish stuck in a fishbowl, looking out onto everyone else who was participating in the *world*, in *life*. I felt completely left out. This isolation, this inability to plan, this feeling invalidated by many around me who couldn't grasp what I was going through—all of this at times led to feelings that did not fit neatly into diagnostic categories of anxiety or depression but certainly contributed to chronic distress that formed the backdrop of my daily experience of caregiving.

An additional and frequently overlooked contributor to psychological burden is resentment. Like Jennifer, many caregivers experience significant resentment because of feeling forced into caregiving, or worse, feeling forced into taking care of someone with whom they have had a difficult relationship. This could include feeling expected to take care of parents who were in the past absent or even abusive to you or caring for partners who you were considering leaving until a life-altering diagnosis came into the picture. Or it could include feeling boxed into a certain job or career that you can't leave because your care partner is on your health insurance plan and leaving that job to meet your needs would mean compromising their medical care. Resentment is a natural reaction to experiencing losses in any aspect of relationships due to illness, such as a loss of a sense of equality, a loss of shared dreams, or a loss of physical intimacy. This was the case for Stephen, the forty-year-old husband and caregiver of Christine, who was being treated for early-stage breast cancer. Before cancer, Stephen and Christine had an exciting sex life, but after treatment—which included a mastectomy of her right breast and oral tamoxifen therapy—Christine lost interest in sex completely. It had been two years since her diagnosis, and two years since they had engaged in any form of physical intimacy. Stephen shared with me that he felt guilty for even thinking about the changes in their intimate life, but at the same time, he acknowledged how this significant change was felt by him as a loss, and he resented her for it. Our work centered on helping him to refocus his resentment and frustration on cancer, not Christine, and on helping him to explore ways in which he could reconnect to feelings of intimacy with Christine while respecting her boundaries.

Whatever the driver, resentment casts a dark shadow on an inherently challenging caregiving role and makes it even more important that you attend to your own mental health needs while taking care of someone else.

A final driver of psychological distress is the challenge of balancing your emotional needs with those of the patient. Helping your care partner to cope with their own fears and anxiety and sadness is an additional responsibility that can weigh heavily on top of your own experience of these same feelings. Many patients struggle with being in the patient role, with receiving help and letting you take care of them. They may also feel guilty for needing your help in the first place, for causing you distress, and for the many downstream ways their illness or limitations may impact your life. Their expression of these feelings can be an added weight for you.

This emotional dance was one my dad and I engaged in for our entire journey as partners in care. He was aware of most of the big and little things I was doing to take care of him, of my fierce advocacy during his hospital stays, and of the ways my life orbited around his needs. Whenever he was lucid, he would make a point when speaking with his healthcare providers to say some version of, "I couldn't do it without her." He wanted me to know that my efforts were valued, even if he was not always conscious of them in the moment when they were happening. His gratitude, however, was accompanied by guilt regarding how much of my time was being taken up by my taking care of him. The enormity of my responsibilities weighed on him, and he frequently expressed feeling guilty about the impact of his needs on my life. In those moments my instinct was always to soothe him and to assure him that I was okay, though I'm confident deep down he knew that wasn't always the case. This balancing act of his navigating gratitude and guilt while I balanced care and burden accompanied us until his death and very much shaped my emotional experience of caregiving.

Physical Burden

In addition to impacting mental health, the burden of caregiving can impact your physical health in both immediate and downstream ways. Caregiving-related injuries can be devastating, and it's surprising that they have received only minimal attention in the scientific literature. Injuries such as pulled muscles, falls, cuts, scrapes, and bruises resulting from care tasks like transferring your care partner from their beds to wheelchairs are more likely to happen when you are worn-out, and when you haven't had the chance to exercise and take care of your body. Not only are these injuries painful but they can limit your capacity to carry out caregiving responsibilities and require your finding additional help, either through a caregiving network of friends and family, or through paid home healthcare workers.

The downstream physical effects of caregiver burden can include difficulty with sleep and fatigue, decreased immune function (notice how you are more prone to colds when you're stressed?), and poor health-related behaviors, such as increased substance use or decreased exercise. As a result of increased stress, you are also at risk for other comorbidities, like hypertension and heart disease, which are common in midlife but made worse by caregiving stress.[24] In fact, one large cohort study of nearly three hundred thousand spousal caregivers of patients with cancer in Sweden found that caregivers had increased risks of coronary heart disease and stroke that persisted over time, and that such risks were particularly high among caregivers of patients with cancers with high mortality rates, like pancreatic, liver, and lung cancers.[25] A study of 1,517 caregivers of cancer survivors in the United States followed for eight years identified high rates of heart disease, arthritis, and chronic back pain several years after initial caregiving experiences,[26] underscoring the long-term health effects of earlier caregiving stress.

One key contributor to these physical effects of caregiving is low healthcare utilization; while caregivers are *experts* at getting their care partners seen by medical professionals, they often are dramatically less successful at doing the same for themselves. Given so many competing demands, caregivers often forgo preventive services and delay screenings and general healthcare follow-ups for themselves. I certainly was guilty of this, and can remember at least one healthcare screening visit that I postponed twice due to my prioritizing my dad's medical needs. Whether or not you identify as a caregiver right now, I want you to take a moment and think about which of your routine medical appointments you have missed or failed to schedule. Why is that? What can you do right now to ensure that these appointments make it to your calendar? Before reading further, I encourage you to make a commitment to taking at least one step toward keeping up with your own healthcare. When we ignore our physical health, when we let little concerns go untreated, we put ourselves at risk for more severe problems later. This risk is never worth taking, especially if you are shouldering the responsibility of taking care of someone else with their own chronic or life-limiting illness.

Like emotional distress, physical burden does not necessarily end with the culmination of your caregiving responsibilities. Without support and attention, high blood pressure worsens, difficulty with alcohol dependence can remain, and significant weight gained during years of intense caregiving responsibilities tends to stay on. This is why taking time for your own medical screenings and check-ups is so important; the stress of caregiving has a significant impact on your body, and that stress can continue to affect you even when your active caregiving journey has ended.

For me, my enduring physical burden took the shape of debilitating exhaustion resulting from chronic insomnia. Insomnia is one of the most common, distressing, and impairing physical concerns for caregivers in the United States.[27] I had experienced sporadic bouts with insomnia years before I became a caregiver, but 2013 solidified my symptoms through classical conditioning. I was on high alert at all times; from countless all-nighters at my dad's bedside in the hospital, to anticipating an emergent phone call in the middle of the night from one of his home health aides, my body eventually unlearned the ability to maintain normal rhythms and sleep at night. I relied for many years on Ativan (a highly addictive antianxiety medication) to help me sleep for even short periods of time at night or for two hours between an all-nighter at the hospital and work, and I eventually added Ativan dependence to my list of caregiving-related effects. Trauma and grief made any attempts to go off Ativan while I was actively taking care of my dad after my mom's death impossible, as did the profound grief I experienced after his death. It was only after the intensity of all the effects of caregiving on me had subsided that I was finally able to tolerate the excruciating physical and psychological pain that is Ativan withdrawal and remove it from my system for good. While I am not ashamed of my Ativan use—it was a survival mechanism—there are other tools that can help you sleep.

These include the powerful cognitive and behavioral strategies[28] that I used to eventually get off Ativan, some of which are discussed in the next chapter.

Financial Burden

A recent estimate indicated that the care provided by family caregivers is valued at six hundred billion dollars.[29] *Six hundred billion dollars!* And yet, this care comes at a significant financial cost to caregivers themselves. Financial toxicity refers to the medical debt and psychological distress patients and caregivers experience due to high out-of-pocket costs of treatment, increased cost-sharing, and decreased household income because of illnesses and treatment. This financial burden resulting from illness and care has been described as having three categories:[30] direct costs, which include the use of financial resources for medical and nonmedical care and the time spent obtaining such care; indirect costs, or the costs that result from a loss of resources or opportunities because of illness; and psychosocial costs, the intangible downstream psychosocial costs that result from illness,[31] such as the downstream costs of psychological burden on patients and families. Direct costs of illness have received the most attention; one large review of studies of the direct costs of cancer care in the United States found that patients and their caregivers spend between $180 and $2,600 each month on care.[32] Such healthcare expenditures are particularly profound for underinsured and underemployed families.[33] In fact, another study[34] found that 70 percent of uninsured patients had catastrophic healthcare expenditures—that is, out-of-pocket health expenses that exceeded 40 percent of their annual income remaining after paying for food.[35]

Systematic evaluations of the financial impact of caregiving are somewhat more limited, but we know that at least one-fifth of American caregivers report high financial strain, and this strain is highest among caregivers between the ages of eighteen and forty-nine[36] and for those who earn $50,000 or less annually. One study found that female caregivers are approximately two and a half times more likely to end up in poverty later in life than their non-caregiving counterparts.[37] Another study calculated the average lifetime loss of $324,000 for a woman leaving the labor force early to care for parents.[38] Not surprisingly, most caregivers report having to depend on savings if they have any, taking out debt, borrowing money from friends, or letting bills go unpaid.

Financial strain can become severe and impact decision-making around medical care. One caregiver I worked with shared considering the risks and benefits of taking her mother off an anticoagulant medication against her physician's advice because paying for the medication meant not being able to put food on the table. Additionally, caregiving often occurs in the setting of other financial difficulties, such as the experience of caregivers taking care of spouses or partners who, because of the effects of their illness or treatment, have had to stop working altogether and have already lost one source of income. This is a particular concern for adolescent and young adult caregivers who had previously been supported financially by parents or guardians but who, because of the effects of illness on work, have lost that financial support. Importantly, the financial impact of caregiving does not end with the cure of an illness or the death of the patient, and in most cases can endure for decades after one's caregiving responsibilities have ended.

Like many caregivers, most of my salary was used to pay for care-related costs, such as the home health aides who took care of my dad, as well as medical supplies, medications, and his food. While peers of mine were spending their twenties and thirties saving and investing money, I often wondered if my paycheck would be able to support my dad's needs. I relied increasingly on credit cards to pick up the slack and learned to say yes to any offers of financial support. As they are for so many caregivers, the economic costs associated with caregiving were high and remain enduring for me. At the same time, I'm aware of how fortunate I was to have had as much financial security as I did; in 2014 when my mom died, I earned over the median family income in the United States. While I struggled to support my dad's medical needs and myself on that income, I know that it would have been dramatically more difficult for me to manage taking care of my dad if I had a lower salary or more limited healthcare benefits for myself built into my employment.

The Burden of Competing Responsibilities

A significant driver of these psychological, physical, and financial components of burden is the challenge of balancing multiple and competing roles and responsibilities. Rarely does caregiving happen in a vacuum; more frequently, caregiving for the medically ill or disabled is superimposed upon other caregiving responsibilities, such as childcare. In fact, approximately nine million Americans are sandwich generation caregivers, providing care for both children and adults.[39] Moreover, 19 percent of Americans are currently providing care to two adults, and 5 percent to three or more adults.[40] Caregivers with multiple caregiving roles have competing demands and more limited emotional, physical, and financial resources to devote to each care recipient. Not surprisingly, then, research has shown that caregivers who provide care to multiple generations at a time have reported worse physical health and less capacity to engage in necessary healthcare services than those who provide care to one adult.[41] Moreover, caregivers who provide lifelong support to a child with intellectual or developmental disabilities while also providing care to an aging parent or other family members are also uniquely at risk for distress.[42] Broadly, as our population continues to age and as the age of first caregiving experience continues to decline, it is anticipated that more and more of you will be caring for multiple individuals at once and therefore at greater risk for the psychological, physical, and financial effects of caregiving.

Trajectories of Burden

Caregiving is predictably unpredictable, and so is the distress you may experience along the way. Burden ebbs and flows, and there is no one common path experienced. Certainly, burden is very much shaped by the presence or absence of an extended family caregiving network, by financial resources, by prior caregiving experiences, and baseline psychological well-being, among many other factors. And yet, we know that when left untreated, distress has the potential to increase across the caregiving trajectory, which is why support can be so beneficial.

There are certain points along this trajectory when distress in caregivers tends to spike. The most obvious time is if treatments stop working and patients transition to end-of-life care, a period when anticipatory grief (that is, grief that occurs before the death of the patient) is often prominent. Paradoxically, caregivers also often experience an increase in distress when patients enter what is called *survivorship*. In oncology, this is a period when patients have completed treatment and may be told that there is no evidence of disease (NED). In other illnesses, such as Lewy body disease, this might be a point after the diagnosis is received and an effective medication regimen has been determined and symptoms stabilize. This is often a point when we see an increase in well-being among patients, who can return to life, albeit to a "new normal." For caregivers, however, this is often the first moment when they can exhale and take stock of everything that has happened. With this exhale often comes a rushing in of anxiety and depression—emotions that may have been avoided during the initial phases of caregiving. Often caregivers will share with me tearfully how they feel like they *should be feeling better* because their care partner is medically stable, but for some reason they feel much worse. I'm guessing some of you may have had this type of experience before. This moment—when you may be feeling a rise in distress despite your care partner doing better medically—is a great moment to reach out for support.

While these trajectories of distress and burden are punctuated at certain moments, they are not predetermined by patient diagnosis or condition, such as cancer versus Alzheimer's disease versus stroke. Certainly, each chronic and life-limiting illness poses unique challenges,[43] such as the changes in cognition and personality that can arise in patients with neurodegenerative diseases like Alzheimer's disease or Lewy body disease or among patients with brain tumors. These symptoms can be particularly devastating to witness and place intense demands on caregivers, as they did for me. But taking care of a loved one recovering from an organ transplant or breast cancer without these illness-driven personality or cognitive changes can be equally as distressing. What is important to keep in mind is that while there are many factors beyond your control that will shape the distress you experience as a caregiver, including elements of your care partner's diagnosis and treatment, there are many other factors, such as your internal emotional resources and your social support system, that can have just as significant an impact on your experience of caregiving. This book explores many of these emotional and interpersonal factors—those that are indeed modifiable—and will give you tools so that you can feel as prepared as possible for the challenges of caregiving, regardless of your care partner's illness and treatment.

Importantly, it's uncommon for caregiving to happen in isolation; it more often co-occurs with other life stresses like job loss or marital difficulties, and is exacerbated in times of large-scale crisis, including natural disasters and war. During the height of the COVID-19 pandemic, caregivers had to, at minimum, shoulder a triple crisis: managing the pandemic, their loved one's illness, and the impact of caregiving on their lives. Added to the typical caregiving responsibilities of assisting patients with their healthcare needs; managing treatment, finances, and care coordination; and providing emotional support was the need to protect loved ones from infection while continuing medical care. While many caregivers took precautionary measures pre-COVID-19 to protect their immunocompromised loved ones, the threat of COVID-19 led to increased measures due to normative fears of infection. For those caregivers who were separated from loved ones receiving care in inpatient settings during the height of the pandemic, engaging in healthcare decision-making and communication with healthcare providers was uniquely challenging and often traumatic,[44] and many caregivers shared that they would choose to sacrifice their own safety to be with their loved ones in these settings. I know I certainly would have felt the same way had my dad been alive.

Combined, these responsibilities contributed to extreme distress and feelings of helplessness.[45] The COVID-19 pandemic severely exacerbated isolation for all of us, but it had particularly devastating effects for caregivers. While historically caregivers have been able to rely on extended caregiving networks of family and friends, as well as on home healthcare workers, during the height of the pandemic, most were providing care in isolation, and many even from a distance. This worsened already-existing social isolation and was especially harmful for older adults whose social networks tend to be already limited.[46] Undoubtedly, the pandemic highlighted how profoundly we rely on caregivers to shoulder tremendous responsibilities, the significant burden they experience as a result, and how important it is that caregivers receive support and resources.

* * *

Are you the only caregiver available to help your loved one? Are other individuals potentially available to help with certain aspects of care, but the majority still falls on your shoulders? This is the reality for many caregivers in the United States. In fact, the majority identify as the primary unpaid caregiver, meaning they are sole caregivers or there are other unpaid caregivers but they themselves provide most of the unpaid care.

This was in many ways the case for me. From the time of that car accident until my mom's death three years later, she and I shared in the day-to-day responsibilities of taking care of my dad. When I received that stomach-dropping phone call from the New Jersey State Police, my mom was at the top of her career. She was not able to focus all her energy on family, which meant that without me to step in, many items on my dad's growing list of medical needs may have gone unattended. Like my patient Jennifer, I felt like there was no choice but to take increasing responsibility for my dad's care. I realized that with this (non-choice) choice I was making many sacrifices, but not stepping in felt impossible for me.

Despite feeling boxed in, however, I realized that I did have some choice in how to capitalize on my—and my mom's—complementary strengths as caregivers and to make the most of our collective care network. You, too, have this choice. Take some time to think through what caregiving responsibilities are easiest for you to accomplish, and which ones can easily be delegated. This type of exercise can help to ensure all caregiving responsibilities are met and mitigate the difficult feelings you may experience if you take on too many of these responsibilities in isolation. For example, perhaps there is someone in your care network who is financially savvy, or who may not be able to handle the day-to-day caregiving tasks but can contribute financially or assist with paperwork and some of the legal aspects of caregiving. Having open discussions about what each of you can, and can't, do will help to prevent disagreements later about who "should have been there." Inevitably, it can help those of you who serve as primary caregivers to feel just a little less resentful of those in your networks who are unable to provide as much hands-on support. And for those of you who are providing care but do not identify as primary caregivers, such discussions can help to clarify the ways in which you can contribute meaningfully to your loved one's care.

My mom and I never had clear communication about our respective roles. This is something I regret, and something I encourage all of you to consider if you are in a similar position. The more we can speak openly about our roles and responsibilities, our strengths and limitations, the more control we can have over our caregiving environment. In Exercise 2.1, I've provided a few talking points that can assist you in navigating this type of conversation with other members of the care network who are involved in some way, however big or small, in caregiving. As you think through these points, it will be helpful to consider the skills you have that may be particularly helpful. For example, if you work in healthcare like I do, you may be more comfortable handling the medical side of things than other family members. Or if you work in finance or law, you may find it easiest to navigate the administrative side of caregiving.

Exercise 2.1: Discussion Points for Navigating Division of Caregiving Responsibilities

- What caregiving tasks will each caregiver be most comfortable doing? Least comfortable? Listing all the necessary tasks can be helpful to answer these questions.
- If you are the primary caregiver, what tasks can be easily delegated to others?
- Does the patient have a preference regarding who assists them with intimate activities of daily living (e.g., bathing, dressing)?
- Having one caregiver serve as the point person for communication with healthcare providers can be beneficial. Who in the care network is best suited to be this person?
- If financial responsibility is to be divided among caregivers, have expectations about financial responsibility been communicated? If not, what's holding you back from having these discussions?
- If one (or more) caregiver(s) is (are) providing care from a distance, what responsibilities can they most reliably accomplish while not being physically present?
- Sometimes patients designate a secondary healthcare proxy. If more than one healthcare proxy has been designated, do all proxies understand the patient's goals of care? Remember, these goals often change across the illness trajectory, so these discussions will need to be repeated.

Instead of having one of these conversations, there was an unspoken agreement between me and my mom, the fine print of which stated that I was my dad's primary caregiver. Perhaps this happened because of how I had navigated the previous few years, or perhaps because of my involvement professionally in healthcare. Unfortunately, my mom and I shared in caregiving responsibilities for only a very short period of time. Her sudden death in 2014 occurred a little over a year after my dad was diagnosed with Lewy body disease. I was in my early thirties and had just joined the faculty at Memorial Sloan Kettering. I had no financial savings and no substantial resources to provide for all the care that my dad needed. I fell into many of the "high risk" categories outlined by the National Alliance for Caregiving.[47] Thankfully, though my bags of material resources were nearly empty, the internal ones were quite full.

CHAPTER 3

A Master Class in Mindfulness

This Magic Moment

Artist: Ben E. King and The Drifters
Arranged and Conducted by Stan Applebaum, 1960

When I meet a caregiver for the first time in clinic, I often share that there is one facet of their experience that is common to all caregivers: uncertainty defines caregiving and sitting with this uncertainty can be extremely challenging. This challenge is present regardless of the site and stage of their loved one's cancer. This challenge is present whether you are taking care of someone with cancer, or dementia, or diabetes, or any other chronic or life-limiting illness, for that matter. Not knowing whether a chemotherapy or a radiation treatment will work leads to uncertainty. Not knowing when your loved one is going to get sick from side effects of treatment leads to uncertainty. Not knowing whether your loved one will be able to communicate after surgery leads to uncertainty. Not knowing if your loved one will be alive in a year, or month, or week, or day, or hour leads to uncertainty. Not knowing if *anything* related to your loved one's care and well-being will impact your ability to accomplish your daily and lifelong to-do lists leads to uncertainty. And for those in bereavement, not knowing when a wave of grief will hit leads to uncertainty. The list is, no doubt, endless.

Feeling a range of emotions during caregiving is expected, and healthy. But to manage these emotions, many caregivers engage in unhelpful coping strategies that lead to extra and unnecessary distress. Here, I want to highlight some areas where you can help yourself to feel a little more in control and ways in which you can live life as fully as possible, despite uncertainty. None of these steps can take away the pain that comes with the thought of a loved one's death, or the loss of being able to achieve certain life goals while being a caregiver. But they can reduce the distress you experience along the way and help you feel stronger. Through this process I'm hoping to empower you to take control of your emotional experience and recognize ways in which your own approach to coping can make an already-difficult experience more challenging.

* * *

My dad had a fanciful imagination and was an extraordinary storyteller, and he used these gifts to write hundreds of children's stories and poems during the last two decades of his life. Because of this part of him, however, when the hallucinations started, it was hard to discern them from what had been, up until his ninety-first year, the products of his whimsical imagination. They started in a subtle way. I would come home after work and my dad would ask when we had gotten the new, brightly colored painting in the living room. He would say that he was seeing art on the wall he had never seen before, but nothing that I could see with my own eyes. Sometimes the hallucinations would be more obvious, such as when he would see small children or puppy dogs running around his bed. I wish I could say that these were pleasurable images, but he shared that none of the children would speak to him, and the dogs wouldn't bark at him or come to him when he called for them. I learned after describing these visions to his doctors that these types of hallucinations, in which the characters are either silent or do not address the individual hallucinating, are a distinctive sign of Lewy body disease, the progressive neurodegenerative disease with which my dad was diagnosed in 2013. When I think about Lewy body disease, I think about taking some of the worst characteristics of Parkinson's disease and combining them with some of the psychotic disorders I studied during my graduate training in clinical psychology. And then furthermore combining them with some of the most complicated and scary medical problems one could imagine, such as when he had sudden drops in blood pressure and body temperature to near-hypothermia levels.

There were days I would come home from work and my dad would turn away in anger when I approached the bed. I would learn from the aide who had been with him that day that he had hallucinated me, all day long, sitting silently at the edge of his bed. His hallucination of me as a daughter who was unwilling to engage with him was the opposite of who I was each moment that I was with him; turning away and ignoring him was not in my emotional repertoire. He was angry at a false perception of apathy on my part while I was doing everything I could to be present for him. Looking back, those were some of the most devastating days for me, when I would try to repair pieces of our relationship that were broken outside the context of my lived reality.

It was also impossible to know how long the hallucinations would last. Sometimes they would be so brief I wouldn't even recognize that they were happening. Other times they would last for a week without a break. Outside of his coming down with a urinary tract infection or having a missed medication dose, it was difficult to predict when he would fluctuate next, and once he began, when the hallucinations would end.

In some ways, I experienced each fluctuation as a mini death; I never knew if it would be irreversible. Coming home and seeing his small pupils, which I quickly learned signaled his beginning to hallucinate, left me with the biggest lump in my throat; then when he would say "I'm back," the greatest joy (while he had little insight into his hallucinating while it was happening, when the fluctuations ended, he did often express awareness that he had returned from a journey of sorts). With each Lewy body disease fluctuation came my own emotional fluctuation through a cycle of grief and sadness to hope and happiness. This cycle repeated itself countless times during my caregiving journey.

Whether your care partner lives with a neurodegenerative disease that leads to fluctuations in consciousness, a cancer that has minimal direct impact on brain functioning, or any other type of illness, inevitably their condition and your experience of caregiving is going to take you on an emotional roller coaster, as each Lewy body disease fluctuation did for me. For many families, there are numerous medical ups and downs, setbacks followed by rebounds in health that are accompanied by a correlate emotional experience in both patients and caregivers. Indeed, most caregivers I've worked with report cycling through a roller coaster of fear and anticipatory grief to hope and relief each time their loved one has a routine scan. These ups and downs can be worsened if healthcare providers are not frank about prognosis, leading, for example, caregivers to do everything they can to search for a cure when one does not exist, or to worry about possibilities that aren't realistically probable. And even in cases when an illness is diagnosed at a late stage without any hope for a cure, uncertainty is nonetheless present. As Dr. Atul Gawande states, "In all such cases, death is certain, but the timing isn't. So everyone struggles with this uncertainty—with how and when to accept that the battle is lost."[1]

Navigating these ups and downs, learning to tolerate such profound uncertainty, will significantly shape your caregiving journey. In fact, your ability to periodically pause and maintain a focus on the present moment while riding this roller coaster will have substantial benefits for you and your care partners.

Understanding Worry and Rumination

Daisy was twenty-eight when she came to see me. She and her wife, Lily, married two years earlier and had recently begun the IVF process to build a family with a sperm donor. They decided that Lily would carry the child, and during one of her follow-up appointments after her egg retrieval, a suspicious lesion was detected on her cervix. Soon after, Lily was diagnosed with an early-stage cervical cancer. Daisy was devasted by the news but grateful that IVF had led to an early diagnosis (the cancer was localized and had not yet had a chance to spread). Lily was treated with surgery, chemotherapy, and radiotherapy. The cancer responded well to the treatments, and they were told that there was a strong chance of her cancer going into remission.

Despite this news, Daisy found that she couldn't concentrate on her work. She ruminated about the past with thoughts like, "If only we had started the IVF process earlier, perhaps she wouldn't have needed chemotherapy," and "I bet that discomfort she felt last September was a sign of the cancer growing. We should have gone to the doctor then." She also felt guilty that they had agreed for Lily to carry a child, and she now worried that the IVF hormones caused the cancer in the first place. Daisy spent significant time worrying about their future together ("If the cancer returns, Lily is going to die, and I am going to be alone") and their possibility of building a family ("We'll never become parents now"). Often, Daisy would find herself tearing up when they cooked dinner together; she imagined cooking for one at some point in the future after Lily had died, despite her standing right there beside her chopping vegetables. Daisy would spend considerable time thinking about Lily's eventual decline and what her death could look like, even though there was no reason at that time to believe she would die from her cancer. When Daisy couldn't sleep, she would look over at Lily sleeping next to her and imagine her not breathing. On some nights Daisy would stay up for hours to be sure Lily's chest was rising and falling with breath. She felt the need to be on high alert for a death that was, realistically, not expected to occur.

*   *   *

What Daisy struggled to do—what we all as humans struggle to do at some point in our lives—is sit with uncertainty. Take a moment and think about the last time you were sitting with uncertainty. What did it feel like in your body? What types of thoughts did you have? What did you do to cope? Did that coping strategy help?

When we are faced with uncertainty, we tend to engage in worry and rumination. When we worry, we have repetitive thoughts about what *could happen* at some future point in time, from a few seconds later to years down the line. When we ruminate, we have repetitive thoughts about what already happened in the past, often with thoughts starting with "I would/should/could have." While initially it may be odd to think about it this way, worry and rumination are strategies we use to feel better in situations that leave us feeling powerless. The act of worrying or ruminating is something we can do, and so we do it to help mitigate feelings of distress. Unfortunately, these efforts to make ourselves feel better have the opposite effect, and instead reinforce our negative emotions. When I asked you to think about the last time you were sitting with uncertainty, do you remember engaging in worry or rumination? My guess is these thought patterns were happening regardless of your awareness of them at the time.

One such period of uncertainty when both partners in care frequently engage in worry and rumination is when patients with cancer have completed treatment and are told that there is no evidence of disease. Despite patients no longer receiving treatment and often no longer identifying themselves primarily as patients, for many cancer survivors and their caregivers, uncertainty remains high and negatively impacts what has the potential to be a period of emotional well-being. For example, both patients and caregivers experience what has been termed *scanxiety*, anxiety that usually arises shortly before undergoing or receiving the results of a periodic routine scan. This scanxiety becomes a regular part of survivorship life for families facing cancer as well as other chronic illnesses, who often share that they live life in three-, six-, or twelve-month intervals between scans and fear that at any moment the illness may return and once again there will be a medical crisis.

Balancing the ability to acknowledge the possibility of illness recurring or progressing and living life in the present fully is one of your tasks as a caregiver. It's a big task, and not an easy one. Each time my dad returned from hallucinating, I never knew how long I had before the next fluctuation would occur. All I knew was that worrying about the next one would detract from the present moment.

Learning to Live with Pink Elephants

As a child of the eighties, I had been familiar with the concept of worry since I grew up reading the Mr. Men series of books by Roger Hargreaves.[2] One of his characters, Mr. Worry, worries about everything. He even worries about worrying, which is a form of what psychologists call *metacognition*. A wizard frees him of his worries, but Mr. Worry's period of relief is short-lived, and he begins to worry about having nothing to worry about. If the wizard had been a clinical psychologist, he would have likely diagnosed Mr. Worry with generalized anxiety disorder, which is characterized by excessive, persistent anxiety and worry about everyday life events. Generalized anxiety disorder affects 6.8 million Americans, or 3.1 percent of the population, in any given year.[3]

During my first few years of seeing caregivers in my practice, I found that many were meeting criteria for the disorder. However, it wasn't that they were worrying indiscriminately, but instead, caregiving created seemingly endless triggers for worry: They worried about how effective their loved ones' treatments would be; they worried about the side effects of those treatments; they worried about what second- or third-line treatments were available in case the current treatment stopped working; they worried about how competently they would be able to perform the medical and nursing tasks asked of them; and they worried about their jobs, their health, and their finances. They worried about almost every aspect of their life that was touched by their loved one's illness in some way. Certainly, these worries made sense since their caregiving roles created an environment of chronic and multidimensional uncertainty. This environment led to intense and often uncontrollable, impairing worry, even in individuals who had no histories of significant anxiety before caregiving. Across hundreds of sessions, the narratives were similar: not being able to plan—for the next year, or even week or day—ahead caused so much distress. Within each caregiver was a strong desire to have a sense of control over their caregiving-shaped lives.

One such caregiver, Ryan, came to see me shortly after his wife, Tina, was diagnosed with advanced non-Hodgkin's lymphoma. She was in her early fifties and had a successful career in real estate. She was active and led a healthy life. The diagnosis was a complete shock to them both. They married in their late thirties and had expected to spend a long future together. Soon after Tina's diagnosis, the medical team shared that the appropriate treatment would be an allogeneic hematopoietic cell transplantation, an aggressive procedure through which Tina would, in effect, be given a new immune system from a donor. The oncologist discussed the risks and benefits associated with transplant, and the potential side effects, which were extensive. The couple asked the medical team what the chance was for a cure of Tina's cancer, and the possibility of it recurring in the future. The answers they received were somewhat unsatisfying, especially to Ryan. They were told that there was a possibility the cancer would come back, but just no way to know what that chance would be.

When Ryan came to me a month after Tina's diagnosis, he described how difficult it was to hear this from her doctors. He longed for a sense of certainty about her—and their—future, certainty that no one could provide. During the first hundred days following Tina's transplant, Ryan struggled to remain focused on the present and spent much of his time thinking about all the possible negative outcomes in the future. He was always on the lookout for signs and symptoms of the transplant not taking and even when Tina looked and felt well, he would get inwardly bombarded by images of her emaciated and dying.

Many caregivers have told me about the various ways in which they coped with all this uncertainty, strategies that had been generally unsuccessful over the long term. For example, to manage worry, Ryan would try to purposefully think more pleasant thoughts, distract himself with work, or have an extra glass or two of wine at the end of hard days. These and other common, but not particularly helpful, coping strategies are outlined below. Perhaps these are strategies that you, too, have used at some point in your life. I know I have. Which means you may know that they don't always work.

Examples of Unhelpful Coping Strategies[4]

- Researching on the Internet/Googling
- Procrastinating
- Worrying/ruminating/perseverating (thinking about something again and again)
- Drinking alcohol or using other drugs
- Denying something is happening
- Withdrawing from friends and family
- Avoiding life activities
- Shutting down/shutting off emotions
- Overeating
- Staying in bed during the day

The strategies that Ryan and other caregivers were engaging in are called *avoidance strategies*. They are things we do to avoid thinking about something that causes distress. Avoidance strategies can include things we physically do to avoid difficult emotions, like engaging in excessive exercise, or cognitive strategies, like trying to not think a certain thought. Avoidance strategies can sometimes work in the short term. But ultimately, they serve to intensify the difficult emotions we're avoiding. In fact, if I tell you right now, *Reader, do not, under any circumstance, think of a bright pink elephant!* What happens?

When we try not to think of something, as Ryan did, sometimes we can get rid of the thought briefly, but eventually it comes back, and often stronger. Whether we try to not think about a bright pink elephant, or in Ryan's case Tina's cancer recurring, or in my case my dad's next Lewy body disease fluctuation, the thoughts do eventually return. Which means that avoidance doesn't work. We engage in avoidance strategies because of our desire to avoid intense negative emotions, to soothe and protect ourselves, but ultimately, these strategies eventually reinforce the same emotions we are trying to avoid.

The negative emotions we try to avoid, such as the distress that results from sitting with uncertainty, result from what we think, not from what is happening at a particular moment. That means that two people can be in the exact same situation, but because of the unique thoughts they are having, they can have drastically different emotional experiences. This idea—that it's not a situation that causes our emotions but what we think of in that situation that causes our emotional experience—is at the heart of one of the most powerful therapeutic techniques: cognitive behavioral therapy (CBT). CBT is an evidence-based therapy used to treat anxiety, depression, post-traumatic stress disorder, substance use disorders, and insomnia, among many other concerns.[5] CBT is powerful because it gives us the tools to invite that pink elephant into the room and cope with the distress that results.

The Power of Cognitive Restructuring

When I was in my last year of graduate school and first started providing care to patients with cancer, I worked with two women who illustrated this idea brilliantly. Both were lung cancer survivors with no evidence of disease who were doing well medically, and both had experienced dyspnea, or difficulty breathing, around the time of their diagnosis. Back then, my office was located on the seventh floor of a building on Beacon Hill in Boston, and each woman had decided to walk up the stairs to our session. The first woman shared with me when she got to our session that despite how winded she felt, she was proud of herself for being able to walk from her apartment to the hospital and then up the stairs. She had become thoroughly deconditioned during her cancer treatment and had begun to regain her strength and stamina in recent months. She was out of breath but reacted to that breathlessness with excitement and pride. The emotion she felt was pure joy. The second woman had also walked to the appointment and up the stairs, but instead of feeling excitement and pride, she felt dread. She shared that she believed that her cancer must be returning; she was out of breath, and that was one of the symptoms that accompanied her lung cancer diagnosis a few years earlier. "The cancer must be back," she thought, feeling pure terror. The two women had drastically different thoughts about being out of breath, and those thoughts contributed to drastically different emotional experiences.

Back then, both women were enrolled in a clinical trial of CBT for anxiety. CBT focuses on altering our interpretation of a stressor—the thoughts we have in potentially distressing situations—to influence the emotional response in the presence of that stressor. This adjustment in thinking is accomplished through what is called *cognitive restructuring*. This process involves identifying thoughts that arise, evaluating how realistic or helpful the thoughts are, and replacing them with ones that are more realistic or helpful. The CBT practitioner highlights unhelpful thought patterns and uses open-ended questions to help patients challenge their thoughts.

Table 3.1 includes examples of common unhelpful thought patterns caregivers have. As you read through, take note of any thought patterns you've had before, particularly those that you've experienced many times in the past. We all engage in these types of thoughts at various times in our life, and we each tend to have a few that are our "favorites," that is, those we have frequently.

Table 3.1: Common Unhelpful Thought Patterns in Caregivers

Thought Pattern	Explanation	Example
All or nothing thinking	You see things in black and white, absolute categories.	*I gave him the wrong medicine; I'm a total failure as a caregiver.*
Over-generalization	You see a single negative event as a never-ending pattern of defeat.	*Something always goes wrong whenever I try to help.*
Mental filter	You dwell on the negatives and ignore the positives.	*The blood work showed no sign of infection or concern, but it doesn't matter at all because he didn't have the energy to walk with me today.*
Disqualifying the positive	You reject positive experiences or successes by insisting they "don't count" for some reason or another.	*The scan results were great, but I'm confident he'll be in the 20 percent of patients whose disease recurs.*
Mind reading	You assume someone is reacting negatively to you, without evidence to support this fact.	*My family doesn't care and has no desire to help.*
Fortune-telling	You anticipate that things will turn out badly and you feel that your prediction is a predetermined fact.	*This will never get easier.*

Thought Pattern	Explanation	Example
Catastrophizing	You attribute extreme and horrible consequences to the outcomes of events.	*Her scan was delayed a week and I'm confident her cancer will spread during that time.*
Emotional reasoning	You assume that your negative emotions necessarily reflect the way things really are ("I feel it so it must be true").	*I have been feeling so overwhelmed lately so I know I'm letting my family down.*
Should statements	You criticize yourself or others with "shoulds" and "shouldn'ts." "Musts," "oughts" and "have tos" are similar examples of self-criticism.	*I should be happier and able to keep it together for my family.*
Labeling and mislabeling	You identify with your shortcomings. Instead of saying, "I made a mistake" and describing an error, you attach a negative label to yourself (e.g., "I'm an idiot" or "I'm a burden").	*I'm totally incompetent, I have no idea how to take his blood pressure.*
Personalization	You see negative events as indicative of some negative characteristic of yourself, or you take responsibility for events that were not your doing.	*My husband didn't get an appointment next week because I'm not aggressive enough with scheduling.*

Cognitive restructuring is a powerful tool and is one of the reasons why CBT is the gold standard therapeutic technique for addressing anxiety and depression.[6] With the first woman, there was very little cognitive restructuring for me to do; her thoughts were helpful and led to her experiencing positive emotions. So instead of cognitive restructuring, I reinforced her feelings of pride and encouraged her to keep track of any thoughts that could indicate a misinterpretation of her physical symptoms. With the second woman, however, we used cognitive restructuring to assist her in recognizing the unhelpfulness of her thoughts.

The process of cognitive restructuring can be boiled down into the following three steps, which you can use to work with any of your own thought patterns that might cause you distress:

Step 1. Identify the thoughts that are associated with difficult emotions, like fear or sadness: The first step is to explore the thoughts you are having when you feel distress. We don't typically go through our days taking stock of our thoughts, so this might feel challenging at first. You might find it helpful to write down whatever comes to mind and then identify the thought that is the most triggering to you. Once you've identified the distressing thought, see if any of the unhelpful thought patterns listed in Table 3.1 are infused in the thought. Often, we can find several unhelpful patterns in the thoughts we have that lead us to feel distress.

For example, with the woman above, we identified the thought "my cancer must be back" as the one that was causing distress, and why she felt this thought to be true (the physical feeling she had after climbing the stairs to my office reminded her of how she felt when her cancer was first diagnosed). We also identified this thought as an example of *catastrophizing*, and she shared that throughout her life she did tend to catastrophize and imagine the worst-case scenarios coming true.

Step 2. Evaluate the evidence supporting the thoughts associated with difficult emotions: Once you've identified the triggering thought, the next step is to evaluate the extent to which you believe the thought to be true. You can do that using the following questions: *What's the evidence that my thought is true/untrue? Is there an alternative explanation? What's the effect of believing this thought? What would happen if I didn't believe this thought?* It can be helpful to write down your answers to these questions using two columns, labeled "Evidence For" and "Evidence Against" to organize your data.

I also encourage you to rate the strength of your belief in your thought, from 0 to 100 percent, as well as the strength or intensity of the distress you feel when you have that thought (again, from 0 to 100). This 0 to 100 rating is called a Subjective Unit of Distress Scale (SUDS),[7] with 0 being no distress and 100 being the maximum amount of distress you can experience. Using the SUDS scale can be particularly helpful in highlighting changes in the intensity of your distress over time as a result of cognitive restructuring.

Using the example of the woman above, we examined any evidence she had that the breathlessness was an indication that her cancer was recurring (she said "none really"), as well as the strength of fear she felt when she had that thought (80 percent).

Step 3. Develop alternative and more helpful thoughts: The final step in cognitive restructuring is to come up with an alternative thought that is more helpful and rational, using the data that you collected during Step 2. It can be powerful to begin the new thought with a statement of validation. For example, with the woman above, she shared the following revised thought: "It makes sense that I feel anxious because the breathlessness reminds me of how I felt when I was first diagnosed, but as of today there is no proof that my cancer has recurred." When you come up with your alternative thought, take note of how it feels to you emotionally to sit with the thought.

My hope is through this process you'll find that your adjustment in thinking leads to a decrease in distress. For my patient, the new thought allowed her to connect to a feeling of hope for her future, instead of dread.

During the period when I worked with these two women, it became clear to me that there was a significant difference between doing CBT with patients with cancer and their caregivers and the graduate students seeking counseling at my doctoral program's outpatient psychotherapy clinic where I was also working: There were many more grains of truth to the catastrophic thoughts caregivers were having (such as "If his cancer returns, he will die") than the students ("I had such a bad headache last weekend, I must have a brain tumor"). The traditional approach of directly challenging the validity of thoughts was not always helpful or even appropriate with patients with cancer and their caregivers, as the illness setting created many realistic concerns related to diagnosis, treatment, and prognosis, and challenging these thoughts could be invalidating and even harmful.[8] I realized early on that to best support patients and their caregivers, it would be necessary for me to work carefully to differentiate negative self-talk that could be realistic (e.g., "If the cancer recurs, his life expectancy will be limited") from unrealistic (e.g., "If his cancer recurs, I will not be able to survive") so that I could be most effective in helping them cope with their lived reality, with their pink elephants.[9]

Given this, to support caregivers struggling with worry and rumination, much of my work focuses on teasing apart the realistic and helpful thoughts from those that are unrealistic or unhelpful. Certainly, we can experience a lot of distress even if our thoughts are realistic. For example, the thought "If the cancer recurs his life expectancy will be limited" might be realistic but it is undoubtedly *very* distressing. If you have a thought like this, there may not be any cognitive restructuring for you to do. Instead, allow yourself to fully express the intense negative emotions that result from having that thought. This is called *emotion-oriented coping*. Take some time to describe, perhaps out loud to a trusted friend or written down in a journal, the range of emotions you feel when you imagine a future without your loved one. Try to articulate as clearly as possible all your concerns about the future and your ability to cope with whatever challenges lie ahead. Through this process, you'll likely find that difficult but rational thoughts are rich opportunities to connect vulnerably to emotions and in so doing, to live in the present moment more fully.

With the example above, after giving space for the expression of emotions, I might encourage you to share how you would choose to spend your time if your loved one's life expectancy is indeed limited, and if there is anything you would do differently. The shift here is not in your thinking but in your behavior, through adjusting how you respond to the limitations in front of you.

Emotion-oriented coping, connecting fully to intense negative emotions, is certainly not comfortable, and it's not something we're necessarily taught to do. However, while sitting with sadness and fear is painful, it's not harmful. It's the opposite approach—avoiding these feelings—that is detrimental to us. Frequently, I sense in my patients a fear of emotions, a fear of feeling intense sadness. In fact, many of the thoughts caregivers share with me are judgments about feelings and thoughts about thinking, or metacognitions, such as "Is it normal that I am thinking this thought? Is it normal that I am feeling so sad?" The answer I almost always give is "Yes!" Emotions are messengers, and it would be strange (and concerning!) to not feel fear or sadness when thinking about a loved one's illness or even death. Making space for these emotions is important and can help you to cope as your caregiving journey unfolds. So instead of hiding that bright pink elephant, I want you to invite it into your room, as my patients do. In fact, it is often in sessions with me that caregivers allow themselves to openly acknowledge their fears of their loved one's death for the first time.

The benefits of this emotional expression are great. I liken it to exercising a muscle. The more you can allow yourself to fully feel intense emotions, the stronger your capacity to tolerate them will be. With each repeated emotional exposure, your emotional tolerance increases. This capacity, or emotional flexibility, allows you to experience intense emotions and then recover, which means that over time, you can feel the full range of feelings that accompany caregiving without great detriment. In so doing, you will be better able to cope with uncertainty, and engage in less worry and rumination. This is why my colleagues and I often use mindfulness-based practices, like meditation, to help caregivers strengthen their capacity to sit with emotions. These practices help us to notice uncomfortable thoughts and associated feelings without reactions like judgment or avoidance.

It's important to note that not every thought you have is completely realistic or unrealistic, but instead it's possible to have thoughts that have parts to them that are both realistic and unrealistic. For example, one caregiver recently said to me, "If I leave work to take care of my mom full time, I'm going to have difficulty keeping up with bills and I'll never be able to secure a job again." The first part of that thought—*I'm going to have difficulty keeping up with bills*—may indeed be true when she stops working. However, the second part—*I will never be able to secure a job again*—is likely unrealistic. With thoughts like these, it's important to first validate the part of your thought that is realistic, that is, acknowledge and give space for the difficult emotions that arise when thinking that thought, before moving on to restructuring the second part of the statement.

Cognitive restructuring is a powerful approach to handling distress, especially when combined with problem-solving. As you go through the process of adjusting your thinking, you might find that the process of gathering data to support or challenge your distress-inducing thoughts might inspire some action on your part, perhaps some step you can take to attend to your needs. When you examine your adjusted thought, consider whether there is something that you can *do* to respond to the thought. If there's something to do, then your job is to do it! This approach is appropriately termed *action-oriented coping*.

Let me illustrate this with a thought I've heard repeatedly in clinic: "If his cancer recurs and he dies, I will not be able to survive." While it's a certainty that coping with the death of a care partner will be difficult, not being able to survive the loss is unlikely. This thought falls into several categories of unhelpful thinking patterns outlined in Table 3.1, such as catastrophizing and fortune-telling. Through cognitive restructuring, one woman who expressed this fear to me was able to share the more helpful thought "I'm scared that I won't be able to survive if my husband dies, but I will do everything I can to take care of myself." This thought then inspired a discussion of action-oriented coping, that is, steps she could take while her husband was alive to enhance the support she would have available in the future so she would feel less alone when he died. I encouraged her to share her fears with close friends and family and to make sure that a plan would be in place to reduce her social isolation after his death.

While it can be incredibly helpful to work with a trained CBT practitioner, this process of working with your thoughts to improve coping is something that you can do on your own. I encourage you to use the following figure[10] to guide you in managing caregiving-related worries:

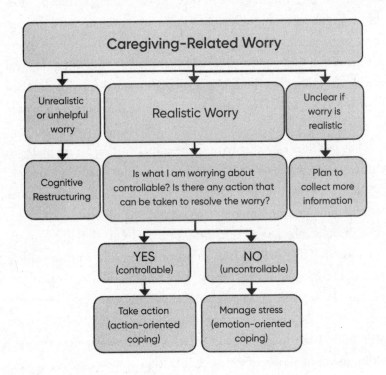

Let me illustrate how you can use this figure yourself. First, determine whether the thought you're having is realistic or unrealistic. If you're not sure, it's important to gather more information so that you can decide. If the thought is unrealistic, engaging in cognitive restructuring can help you to come up with a more rational and helpful thought. If the thought is realistic, however, and it's nonetheless associated with distress, the next step is to figure out whether there is any action you can take in response. For example, many caregivers are worried about talking to their loved one about what treatment options might be available in the future. The thought

"I'm worried that talking to my husband about what might happen if this treatment stops working is going to really upset him" might be realistic *and* distressing. However, through opening the conversation with her husband, a caregiver with this thought may find that her husband is relieved to have the conversation because it's been weighing on him as well. Finally, if the distressing thoughts you are having are realistic and uncontrollable (meaning, there is no action to take), then the best approach is to engage in emotion-oriented coping, that is, to allow yourself to fully feel and express the emotions that arise.

The next time you find yourself stuck in a cycle of worry, see if you can use this diagram to help you cope more effectively and productively with your thoughts.

I want to make it clear that none of these changes in thinking happens overnight. Your thoughts are not like a light switch that you can just turn on and off; if they were, I'd be out of a job. Instead, adjusting your thinking involves a deliberate process over time. It takes effort, but the payoff can be huge: You can use each period of uncertainty as an opportunity to examine unhelpful thoughts, to develop new coping strategies, and to allow for vulnerable emotional expression. Together, this is a major exercise in resilience. If with each cycle of worry and rumination you can begin to engage in this process, over time you can expand your capacity to navigate uncertainty without added negative emotions. You can strengthen your internal muscle and develop tools to help you move through your caregiving journey without significant detriment to yourself. Through this lens, you can choose to capitalize on the challenges of caregiving and use them to develop strength, resilience, and the capacity for more mindful living.

The Practice of Letting Go

This idea of sitting with uncertainty, of capitalizing on these moments as opportunities to develop new strengths, is certainly not novel. It's an idea that underlies much of Buddhist thought and practice, which I immersed myself in soon after my mom's sudden death in 2014 through the writings of Pema Chodron. Chodron's words guided me to learn to tolerate waves of intense emotional pain, to sit quietly with uncertainty, and to recognize my role in making periods of uncertainty worse through my incessant worry. I by no means have become an expert at this, but I now recognize how overpowering my thoughts can be and have learned to let go of needing to respond to them. In *The Age of Dignity*, Ai-jen Poo reflects on the writings of Pema Chodron in her discussion of facing death:

> Chodron writes, "We are raised in a culture that fears death and hides it from us. Nevertheless, we experience it all the time. We experience it in the form of disappointment, in the form of things not working out. We experience it in the form of things always being in a process of change. When the day ends, when the second ends, when we breathe out, that's death in everyday life." That means we have endless moments to practice letting go, to learn about grieving and to prepare for death.[11]

Caregiving provides vast opportunities to practice letting go, which means that you will have endless moments to strengthen your capacity to do so and to live a richer, more mindful life. Each time you receive disappointing medical news about your loved one is a chance to let go. Every moment that a loved one expresses suffering is a chance to let go. Each time you leave your loved one's side in the hospital is a chance to let go. Every moment you witness a physical change in your loved one is a chance to let go. Each time you say good night to your loved one is a chance to let go. Every one of these moments is an opportunity to strengthen your capacity to let go, and to choose to live life more fully.

When I speak about the idea that caregiving is an opportunity for growth, I often reflect on the words of another Buddhist teacher and psychologist, Dr. Tara Brach, whose lectures have become a regular part of my Saturday morning routine. "Metacognition is our superpower," she often says. "We can observe and recognize thinking."[12] Learning to notice when you engage in cycles of worry, examining the accuracy and helpfulness of your thoughts, and allowing yourself to connect to sadness when present and appropriate—these are all strengths. These are all indeed superpowers. Caregiving provides you with countless opportunities to cultivate this superpower. Each time you take note of ways in which your unhelpful thought patterns are making already-challenging situations more difficult, that is a superpower. Each time you allow yourself to fully feel intense but appropriate emotions—like sadness and fear—without avoidance, that is a superpower. It's no surprise, then, that time and again I hear from caregivers about how caregiving engendered within them feelings of resilience and strength they were not aware of before. Caregiving gave them powers they never knew before.

Nina was one such caregiver. Her husband, Harry, underwent a long and arduous treatment for esophageal cancer that began with surgery and was followed by chemotherapy and radiation. When Harry was first diagnosed and scheduled for surgery, Nina was not sure if he would survive what was ahead, and throughout his treatment she rode a steep roller coaster of uncertainty. A year and a half later, Harry completed treatment, and for a brief moment, Nina was hopeful about the future. This period of well-being was short-lived, however, because Harry suffered a heart attack a month later. In session with me, Nina shared intense shock and devastation at what she perceived to be a downstream effect of the cancer treatment on Harry's heart, and a belief that a full recovery was now impossible. Our work together during this time focused on helping Nina to process the intense fear and sadness she was feeling, and to highlight how she had previously coped so successfully with uncertainty. This uncertainty accompanied her as Harry slowly recovered, first in the hospital and then at a subacute rehabilitation center. Two years after his initial diagnosis, Harry returned home completely physically deconditioned but medically stable with no evidence of cancer in his body.

Harry's return home coincided with New York City going into lockdown at the outset of the COVID-19 pandemic. During one of our first sessions during that time, Nina shared with me a feeling that suddenly a torrent of negative emotions seemed to come crashing down on her. It was almost as if as soon as she knew that her husband was okay, it was okay for her to not be okay. Nina felt worn-out, like she had run an ultramarathon, and instead of putting her at a finish line that would allow for freedom, Harry's recovery coincided with the beginning of the pandemic, and extended what had already been an enduring period of challenge to one that ultimately became forty-plus months long.

What stands out to me about Nina, though, was her ability to feel an immense sense of strength despite being so worn-out. She shared that the uncertainty she and her husband faced during his cancer treatment and heart attack had ultimately prepared them for the pandemic. In fact, she told me that facing the added challenges of COVID-19 was "nothing compared to his illness!" What *was* challenging was the prolonged period of isolation brought on by the pandemic, serving to delay further their plans to travel and reconnect with family and friends. But she believed that caregiving, and particularly learning to sit with profound uncertainty during his multiple medical challenges, helped her to feel stable and grounded and prepared emotionally for the added challenges brought on by the pandemic. In this regard, she was able to see that she was coping better than her non-caregiver friends. Nina was able to connect to a growing sense of appreciation of her strength and unique perspective that had been developed and reinforced during her months of intense caregiving.

The Power of Calming Our Bodies

This capacity to reflect on uncertainty in caregiving as an opportunity for growth is not an idea I would suggest if you're in crisis or newly in the role. In these moments, even gentle cognitive restructuring or action-oriented coping can feel challenging. If you are one such caregiver, there are other, more immediate stress-management strategies that I want you to use, such as those that focus on your physical feelings. Every emotion has three components to it: *a thought* that is often the driver of emotions, as explored previously; *a behavior*, which often falls into the category of unhelpful coping strategies discussed earlier; and a *physical feeling* that accompanies the emotion, such as a racing heart or tightness in your shoulders. This means that we have three ways to cope with difficult emotions: adjustments to our thinking such as through cognitive restructuring, adjustments to our behaviors, and adjustments to our physical feelings.

Focusing on the physical feelings that accompany difficult emotions is a powerful place to start, especially in moments of high stress.

One of the most effective ways to address how we feel physically is through our breath. *Diaphragmatic breathing* is a consistently powerful stress-management tool available to us, and at the end of this chapter, I provide an overview of how to practice this technique. You can practice diaphragmatic breathing in almost any circumstance (except for those where practicing would be dangerous, such as when you're driving). Taking deep diaphragmatic breaths before difficult conversations with your care partner, before appointments with a doctor, or before making a big decision can have a positive impact on how you feel emotionally and how you subsequently handle these experiences. Ultimately you may find that your breath becomes the most accessible and consistently successful emotion-oriented coping strategy available to you.

Since every emotion has a physical component to it, calming your body can directly target emotions like anxiety. In fact, I taught diaphragmatic breathing to the two women I introduced you to earlier in the chapter who had different interpretations of being out of breath. Since the second woman misinterpreted the physical symptom of breathlessness as a sign her cancer had returned, diaphragmatic breathing helped her to not only calm her body but prove to herself that this symptom was in fact under her control, and not associated in the present moment with cancer.

There are many other stress-management techniques in addition to diaphragmatic breathing that can calm your body (as well as your mind), such as progressive muscle relaxation, body scans, and yoga. Since each of us is unique, some of these approaches may feel more helpful to you than others. Take some time to figure out which approach is easiest and most effective for you, and then see if you can integrate it into your stress-management routine. I encourage you to try practicing your chosen approach at least twice a week, though of course daily practice is ideal. You'll likely find that even just five minutes of practice a day can eventually make a big difference in how you feel.

*   *   *

In April of 2013, my dad was given an antipsychotic medication to address worsening delirium that came on while he was being treated for a urinary tract infection in the ER, and this dose put him into a coma. The silver lining is this coma gave his team of neurologists the hint that he might have Lewy body disease. That period while he was in the coma, however, was one of the most painful for me emotionally.

I remember walking home from the hospital one night, with tears streaming down my face as I listened to all the voice messages he had left me that I had saved on my phone. I had no idea if I would ever hear him speak again. His body was still here, but he wasn't. I was swimming in a deep sea of uncertainty. I went through those days with my stomach in my throat. I tried to practice the cognitive restructuring and diaphragmatic breathing techniques I've shared with you in this chapter. I found it so hard to take those deep breaths, though I continued to practice daily. I quickly realized that my breath was one of the few things I had control over. I couldn't avoid the painful emotions, which came in torrential waves. I did a lot of crying, a lot of talking to him, and holding his hand and rubbing his feet. I tried to remain present and not go down the path of imagining his funeral and how life would look after his death. It was a crash course in sitting with uncertainty that ultimately ended a few weeks later when an effective medication was administered, and his right eyelid started to open—just a sliver—and then his left.

After he emerged from the coma and began formal treatment for Lewy body disease, my dad's cycling in and out of fluctuations of consciousness became a regular part of life. Each cycle connected me to the feelings I had when he was in the coma, but I found myself with each cycle a bit better able to cope with the uncertainty. I lost count of the number of times my dad fluctuated between 2013 and his death in 2019, though my guess would be upwards of fifty. Each cycle not only cultivated my capacity to tolerate distress but also intensified what had already been an incredible appreciation for moments when he and I could connect, even if briefly. It was this capacity that allowed me to accompany him with complete presence during some of his most difficult moments, including his four-day stay in the ICU before his death. Those first two days he was lethargic and spent most of his time sleeping, but on the third morning, when he was energized from IV hydration, antibiotics, and actual sleep, I sat down next to him and scratched his head, and he opened his eyes and said, "Baby doll, let me give you a hug." The tangled wires of the heart monitor on his chest made it tricky for him to open his arms, but eventually I found my place on his shoulder. I could feel his heartbeat under mine. I was fully present. My years of coping with uncertainty had allowed me to completely forget about the surroundings and be fully in that moment. Working through the cycles of uncertainty allowed me to relish what was the last time he opened his arms to hug me.

Figure 1. Diaphragmatic Breathing[13]

One of the most powerful and readily-available stress-management techniques that you can use when the demands of caregiving become overwhelming is diaphragmatic breathing. During normal day-to-day activities, and especially during stressful moments, we tend to engage in "chest breathing," taking shallow and constricted breaths. Diaphragmatic breathing, on the other hand, involves much deeper breaths that allow for a full oxygen exchange. This type of breathing slows our heartbeat and lowers our blood pressure, creating a state of relaxation.

Diaphragmatic breathing includes the following steps:

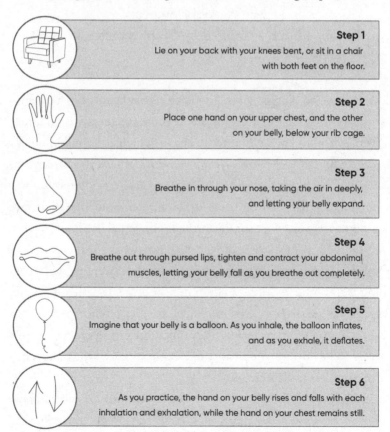

Step 1
Lie on your back with your knees bent, or sit in a chair with both feet on the floor.

Step 2
Place one hand on your upper chest, and the other on your belly, below your rib cage.

Step 3
Breathe in through your nose, taking the air in deeply, and letting your belly expand.

Step 4
Breathe out through pursed lips, tighten and contract your abdonimal muscles, letting your belly fall as you breathe out completely.

Step 5
Imagine that your belly is a balloon. As you inhale, the balloon inflates, and as you exhale, it deflates.

Step 6
As you practice, the hand on your belly rises and falls with each inhalation and exhalation, while the hand on your chest remains still.

CHAPTER 4

Combating Ageism
and Other Forms of Discrimination

I Can Tell The Way You Say Hello

Artist: Paul Hampton
Produced and Arranged by Stan Applebaum, 1962

Discrimination. Stigma. Bias. Prejudice. These factors too frequently shape our experience of healthcare. If you have already been a caregiver, you may have witnessed ways in which discrimination impacted the care your loved one received. Perhaps it was obvious, such as a healthcare provider expressing very clear opinions about your loved one based on some irrelevant attribute, like their race. Or perhaps it was more subtle, through nonverbal behaviors, such as avoiding eye contact. As a caregiver, you may have also experienced how discrimination impacted the way that you were treated. None of us is immune to discrimination in healthcare. Whether it is based on age, race, sexual orientation, gender identity, physical or cognitive capacity, or any other factor, discrimination can negatively impact access to healthcare, the quality of healthcare received, and eventually, countless healthcare outcomes.

While there are efforts to educate healthcare providers about how to best meet the needs of diverse caregivers,[1] more limited attention has been given to ways you can address stigma and discrimination that may be impacting your efforts as a caregiver. However, a foundation of all effective approaches is establishing open communication and advocacy for your needs and those of your care partner. If discrimination takes the form of direct verbal statements, I encourage you to *always* speak up and share your perspective. If it occurs in more subtle ways, such as through nonverbal behaviors, you can use some of the communication techniques I discuss in this chapter to address these behaviors in the moment. Importantly, if healthcare communication is occurring in English but that is not your native language and members of the healthcare team assume you understand what is being stated, ask them to speak slowly and clearly and to explain each medical term used. And if that isn't sufficient, it is your right to ask for a medical interpreter so that you can fully understand what is being said.

Of all the forms of discrimination, my dad's and my experience as partners in care was profoundly shaped by ageism. Ageism is defined as stereotypes, prejudice, and discrimination toward people because of their age. Ageism can be directed at individuals in any age group, but the impact is most detrimental to those who are older adults. In fact, ageism has been identified by the World Health Organization as a global threat to older people's health and well-being.[2] Here in the United States, we're on track to have the largest generation of older adults in human history,[3] whose care will be left to family caregivers.[4] As we age, the number of medical conditions we live with—and our need for healthcare-related support—increases. Given this, it's not surprising that nearly half of caregivers are providing care for individuals with multiple comorbidities,[5] many of whom are older adults with long-term physical conditions and memory problems.

Against this backdrop, many of you will likely provide care for an older adult at some point. Working against assumptions made about your care partner's capacity to live a meaningful life based on their age requires you to be fully aware and informed of the subtle—and not-so-subtle—ways that ageism can shape care delivery. In this chapter, I use our experience of ageism to illustrate how discrimination can impact patients and caregivers, and provide tools for you to recognize and combat it early on. My hope is that I can help empower you to proactively head off and address *any* type of discrimination you or your care partner may encounter.

*   *   *

My dad never let his age stop him from living life to its fullest. In his early seventies, he was entering a new and exciting phase of his career as the principal arranger and orchestrator for the New York Pops, and my brother and I kept him active and running around. He was like the Energizer Bunny through his late eighties. He ate up each moment of life, and never let his chronological age dictate what life should look like. As he neared ninety and his body started to slow down, he struggled to balance continuing to live life fully and accepting a small number of physical limitations. But he made appropriate adjustments that enabled him to be as engaged as possible, and he didn't self-identify as "old" until the last several years of his life.

I learned quickly, however, that the year of birth (1922) listed on my dad's hospital identification bands was often a potential threat to the care he received. From his very first hospitalization until his last year alive, I found myself repeatedly defending the value of my dad's life and his capacity to continue to live a meaningful life. Assumptions were made about what type of life my ninety-something-year-old dad was able to live, what meaningful life meant for him, and what his goals of care should be, according to many of the healthcare professionals who asked us about them. Our experiences were significantly punctuated by discrimination based on the fact that, according to the date of birth on his hospital wristband, he was old. *Old* old, in fact. The concept of "old age" is vague, with definitions ranging from the over-fifties to the over-eighty-fives. Subcategories of old have even been created, including the *young* old (sixty-five to seventy-four), the *middle* old (seventy-five to eighty-four) and the *old* old (eighty-five years and older).[6]

I've lost count of the number of times it felt like the value of my dad's life was questioned by staff, times when it seemed like the care he was receiving was colored by ageism. The most overt experience occurred in 2013 when I had first brought him into the hospital for treatment of a UTI. Two days into the stay he developed delirium, a confused and disoriented mental state that can be triggered by the dysregulation of daily rhythms that occur in the hospital through spending days in an emergency department where the lights are always on. Delirium is common in older adults, in many cases is preventable, and in most cases is treatable. A medical resident came to examine him and then asked to speak with me in the hallway. He had not met my dad before that evening and therefore had not yet had the chance to engage in a meaningful conversation with him. The exchange went something like this:

Dr.: Ms. Applebaum, your dad is very confused.

Me: Yes, I know. It came on yesterday. I had suggested to the team when he was admitted to give him the bed near the window to help resolve the delirium. The lack of light seems to trigger this.

Dr.: Ms. Applebaum, your dad is an elderly man. He's ninety-one.

Me: Yes, he recently celebrated his birthday.

Dr.: I'm reading in the chart, this is his second or third UTI this year, he seems to be getting them repeatedly.

Me: His urologist has been speaking with us about his getting a suprapubic catheter, so that the pain of the Foley insertion could be avoided and he could have better protection against these UTIs.

Dr.: You want to put your father through a procedure?

Me: What we understood is that it is a simple procedure that can be done here during this admission, and which could really improve his quality of life and give him more of his life back. And it's not about me putting him through anything. It's about him still having choice in this matter.

Dr.: Ms. Applebaum, your father is unable to make choices right now.

Me: Exactly. He's delirious. But two days ago he wasn't, and we spoke about the catheter. My dad's UTI is under control. Once the delirium resolves I hope you'll be able to meet him.

Dr.: If my father were ninety-one, I wouldn't be putting him through any of this.

Me: That's my father in that room, and his age doesn't matter here; he's deserving of care no matter how old he is.

This interaction is marked in indelible ink in my mind, as it was the first of what would become many in which the value of my dad's life—and the value of certain medical interventions focused on improving his *quality* of life—was equated with the date of birth listed on his hospital wristband. Indeed, almost every day that he was in the coma, at least one member of the rotating healthcare team would make a comment implying that it would be best to stop treating him with statements like "He's in his nineties, he's had a good life." Yes, my dad was in his nineties and he had had a good life, but that didn't mean that he was ready for his life to end. As I sat by his side during those weeks, I was constantly on the defensive. Their comments made me feel judged, belittled, and small.

In addition to patients being recipients of ageism, ageism can also be "self-directed," that is, through patients' own refusal of certain treatments or procedures. For example, some patients won't seek out care because they assume that certain symptoms are the result of normal aging;[7] in other instances, patients will perceive themselves as too old to be eligible for interventions that could be highly effective. Unfortunately, I've witnessed how this self-directed ageism led to cancers being diagnosed at late stages. Such was the case for Kelly, an eighty-six-year-old woman with advanced melanoma who chose to not see her internist because she assumed based on her age that she was ineligible to have a very visible and palpable lesion removed surgically. Instead, she did nothing, and it was only when the cancer spread to her lungs that she began receiving medical care, at a time that was ultimately too late to be lifesaving.

The association between discrimination, such as ageism, and adverse health outcomes is well established. Among older adults, studies have found that discrimination is associated with poor mental[8] and physical health,[9] decreased informativeness of interactions with healthcare professionals,[10] decreased use of preventive health services[11] such as mammography and colonoscopy,[12] and delays in testing, treatment, and filling prescriptions.[13] Importantly, older adults in receipt of Medicare are less likely to use preventive and necessary medical care in part due to financial concerns related to reimbursement rates and higher out-of-pocket costs.[14] Additionally, underutilization of healthcare services of all kinds by older adults is associated with challenges in securing transportation to and from medical appointments.[15] As such, many older adults do not have the *choice* to receive healthcare that they need and must contend with ways our healthcare system systemically challenges their engagement in care.

These negative effects are amplified when ageism and racism intersect.[16] Racially and ethnically minoritized older adults are more likely to delay or forgo medical care, are disproportionately excluded from medical research, and have increased poor outcomes including disability and death.[17] Similarly, sexual and gender minority older adults experience health disparities,[18] are disproportionately underinsured,[19] and are at particular risk for receiving inequitable healthcare, including palliative and end-of-life care.[20] These outcomes are driven largely by discrimination and rejection from biological families, communities, and society.[21] Indeed, homophobia and transphobia, in addition to structural racism and ageism, ableism, and classism,[22] have long contributed to healthcare disparities and disproportionate rates of death. These disparities were dramatically amplified by the COVID-19 pandemic, which highlighted the intersection of ageism with racism, heterosexism, and transphobia in healthcare.[23]

All these factors contribute to poor outcomes for patients, caregivers, and their extended family networks. While the necessary collective and systemic change to combat ageism and all other forms of discrimination will take time and very purposeful efforts,[24] being informed and aware of the subtle and not-so-subtle ways discrimination presents itself and learning to respond effectively is a big step toward change.

*   *   *

In my early work with patients with cancer, many adults over eighty shared with me a strong conviction that they had lived a full life and were at peace with the idea of their life coming to an end. My dad, on the other hand, felt that his age was not a worthwhile indicator of his future potential and at ninety hoped to live another ten years. There is no one "correct" viewpoint on age. What is important for you as a caregiver, however, is to understand the value your partner in care places on age, whether they look at it as a meaningless representation of chronology or as a meaningful indicator of what lies ahead. This clear understanding will allow you to advocate for care that respects their beliefs about age and their goals for life as a result, whatever that means to them.

While our formal journey as partners in care began when my dad was in his early nineties and ended a week before his ninety-seventh birthday, I don't think our experience would have been drastically different had he been ten, or even fifteen, years younger. Over the past decade, I've heard countless stories in which the care received by patients who were significantly younger than my dad was perceived to be impacted by age-related discrimination.

Lucy, forty, was one such caregiver who came to see me in the fall of 2016. She was an only child whose mother had died of metastatic breast cancer when she was fourteen. Lucy was the only family member or friend available to take care of her father, Tom, who had been diagnosed with advanced prostate cancer. Lucy lived about fifteen minutes away from Tom with her husband and three-year-old son. She worked as a public defense attorney and had a demanding job. Her husband had been recently laid off from his job in healthcare administration, and they had been completely dependent on Lucy's salary for the past eight months. The news of her father's cancer and her new caregiving responsibilities was a significant source of distress for her. When Tom received his diagnosis, Lucy and her father had a lukewarm relationship; she shared with me that she had held on to resentment of him since her mother's death. At that time, Tom was so overwhelmed with grief that he was unable to be emotionally present for her in the way that she needed, and generally unable to parent her. And he expected her, at age fourteen and deep in her own grief, to take responsibility for all the household chores, the "women's work" in the house. Their relationship was tense throughout Lucy's high school years, though it improved once she moved out. When Tom initially reached out for help, Lucy felt resentful that now she was being asked to provide care to the same person who had deprived her of care when she needed it most.

Tom was seventy-eight when he was diagnosed with advanced prostate cancer. He had led a relatively healthy life and was surprised by the diagnosis. He had smoked cigarettes socially in his early adulthood but stopped when he married Lucy's mother, and there was no family history of cancer that he was aware of. He hadn't, however, always kept on top of his medical care. He was a veteran of the war in Vietnam and gotten most of his medical care through the VA system. He received annual notices reminding him to come in for a physical but often ignored them. Each time he did bring himself to the VA, he perceived that the concerns he shared with his doctor were brushed off as signs of "normal aging." This included what he described as an increased urge to urinate during the night and generally feeling like his ability to empty his bladder was decreasing. Tom was seventy-three when he first expressed these concerns, but it was not until two years later that he had a prostate-specific antigen (PSA) test done, which detects a protein produced by both cancerous and noncancerous tissue in the prostate. By the time Tom's cancer was detected, it had already spread to his lungs.

Tom had begun treatment through the VA, but Lucy felt the care he was receiving was suboptimal. She reflected on how long it took for the PSA test to be completed and feared that he was being unfairly dismissed by his physicians as less deserving of medical interventions, perhaps because of his age, or perhaps because he was Black. Additionally, her father had attended the first few appointments on his own but found that he often couldn't understand what his doctors were saying and was fearful of asking questions. He didn't want to appear "dumb."

Lucy attended the subsequent meeting with the oncologist, who shared his concerns about pursuing any form of non-palliative (that is, curative) treatment for Tom. He asked what Tom's goals were for his life, and the tone he used, according to Lucy, was condescending and judgmental. She described her father being spoken to in a manner that implied that he could not have any good reasons to engage in care that could potentially extend his life. The oncologist emphasized the side effects and potential risks of the treatment and seemed to infuse his own judgment about what was "right" for Tom into his clinical recommendations. It was at that point that Lucy was adamant about transferring Tom's care to another facility and sought support from me. When we first met, she spoke about feeling like her father's diagnosis was unnecessarily delayed and that if he was younger, or White, his symptoms perhaps would have been taken more seriously. She felt their current situation was a direct result of the intersectionality of his age and race. In our initial sessions, I focused on supporting Lucy around these painful—and likely valid—cognitions and encouraged her to express her deep anger and sadness. I also highlighted the powerful ways in which she chose to take control over his healthcare in the context of discrimination when she transferred his care away from the VA.

During our second month working together, Lucy shared that her involvement in Tom's cancer care connected her to feelings of longing for their connection to be improved and she felt urgency to repair their relationship given her realization that her time with her dad was limited. Our work subsequently focused on helping Lucy to make the most of the time they had together, including encouraging her to share her regrets with Tom and sadness about the past, and to create new—and happier—experiences together with him in the present.

Studies have found that older patients with cancer like Tom are less likely to be offered standard cancer treatments or participation in clinical trials,[25] due in part to age limits set on trial participation. Moreover, when clinical trials are offered to older adults, they often do not include outcomes that are pertinent to the older adult population, such as preservation of function, cognition, and independence.[26] As such, older adults with cancer are not only the recipients of individual ageist behaviors but systemic ageism. Such experiences no doubt extend to other illness populations.

You are likely familiar with the Golden Rule: *Do unto others as you would have them do unto you.* For healthcare professionals, following the Golden Rule means striving to provide care for patients that is in line with the care that such healthcare professionals would want in similar circumstances. The Golden Rule asks providers to answer the question, "If I were the patient, how would I want to be treated?" and completely leaves out the perspective of the patient. The Golden Rule is what that medical resident was following when he suggested that it was inappropriate for my dad to have a suprapubic catheter inserted, based on what he would do if his father was ninety-one and in the same medical condition. Dr. Harvey Chochinov writes:

> The Golden Rule has its limitations, as it requires some overlap between how we see ourselves and how others see themselves. So long as the patient's values and priorities align with our own, we can infer their needs based on how we would want to be treated in their situation. The more our worldview and lived experience deviates from theirs, the more the Golden Rule begins to unravel. How would I want to be treated if I were that old? If I were that dependent? Or that disabled, dis-

figured, marginalized, or disease ridden? Our own biases and perceptions of current, and the possibility of future, suffering can lead to attitudes that are tone deaf and decisions that are discordant with patients' perceptions, values, and goals.[27]

When healthcare professionals follow the Platinum Rule, *Do unto patients as they would want done unto themselves*,[28] it is more likely that the care that is delivered honors and respects the values and goals of the patient. Following the Platinum Rule requires that healthcare professionals do what Dr. Holland told me they needed to do to truly take care of my dad: They needed to learn about who he was and what mattered to him. To follow the Platinum Rule, healthcare professionals need to know their patients so that they can truly take care of, and care for, them. Looking back, most instances in which it felt to me like my dad's care was colored by ageism were likely instances in which healthcare professionals were following the Golden Rule, not the Platinum Rule.

Combating Ageism the Moment It Happens

So how might you know when ageism is occurring? Sometimes it's incredibly subtle, and sometimes it's obvious. The way members of the healthcare team communicated with my dad was one of the most striking and clear forms of ageism. Frequently they would speak too fast, or not loud enough, or in "elderspeak,"[29] the patronizing tone that includes frequent repetition of questions, inappropriate references (such as referring to my dad as "sweetie"), and collective pronoun substitutions that give the message that the older adult is unable to act independently (saying, for example, "Let's go to the bathroom" or "Are we ready for bed?"). Elder-speak also often includes requests that ask a question but indicate a desired response ("You're ready for dinner now, aren't you?"), and reflective speech that is manipulative, conveys dependence, and controls behavior by encouraging patients to complete tasks ("Take this pill for me"). Paradoxically—due to the higher tones of speech used—elderspeak makes it *more* difficult for speech to be understood. And, undoubtedly, it can be seen as condescending and disrespectful,[30] it promotes dependency,[31] and it increases the probability of resistance to care.[32] In sum, elderspeak poses a threat to patients' dignity.

A broader issue that impacts patients of all ages is when a healthcare team member uses words or phrases that most individuals would not understand, like *ejection-fraction* or *creatinine clearance*. This can intensify the emotional distance between the patient and those who provide medical care and can make it intimidating for patients and caregivers to ask providers to explain what they are saying.

In moments like these, I encourage you to ask questions to check your care partner's understanding, as well as clarifying questions of the healthcare professional. For instance, I would ask my dad, "Did you understand what Dr. Stein just said?" to give him an opportunity to gain clarity. I would make a point to follow up with the healthcare professional by saying, "Dr. Stein, can you explain a bit more about what you mean by that?" or "What does [insert medical term] mean?" These types of questions will help to ensure that no important information is missed.

While I was lucky to have had a lot of experience communicating with healthcare teams, not everyone is comfortable expressing confusion, and this has nothing to do with age. Speaking with medical professionals can be overwhelming and anxiety provoking. Try to challenge yourself to speak up as much as possible to ensure that everything that the medical team is communicating is understood completely by your loved one, and by you.

Some of the anxiety we have when speaking with healthcare professionals is driven by power dynamics that can be exacerbated by certain behaviors, such as physicians talking "at patients" while standing over them while they remain in bed. This is one way that discrimination of all kinds can manifest in healthcare interactions. This frequently happened when my dad was in the hospital and prevented him from maintaining eye contact with his providers and feeling engaged in whatever communication was occurring. This simple dynamic, of the standing physician and bedbound patient, leads to a dramatic power differential that can lead to anxiety, fear, and intimidation in patients and not surprisingly has been shown to have a significant and negative impact on their satisfaction, compliance with medical care, and rapport with the healthcare professional.[33]

Each time I witnessed this happening, my role in helping my dad to engage in healthcare communication came into sharper focus. What I tended to do, when it was physically possible, was stand either behind, or to the far side of, my dad's hospital bed when the medical team rounded so that I was mostly or completely out of my dad's view. I wanted him to have the opportunity to speak directly to the medical team, to take control of the interactions whenever possible, without my presence shaping his responses. The role I assigned myself was that of an ad hoc interpreter; if my dad couldn't hear or understand what was being asked of him, I would step in and repeat the words clearly and slowly. My goal was not to take charge of the communication but to give him the support he needed to be fully engaged. Certainly, there were times he would ask explicitly for me to join in the conversation and times when he couldn't communicate at all, but I generally strived to have him, at a minimum, answer on his own the rounding team's initial questions regarding how he was feeling, how the night went, and what his concerns were at times when he was awake and clearheaded.

How can you assist your loved one in communicating with the medical team and work against ageist behaviors that may be emerging? Have you used any of the approaches that I once did? Any ways in which you can help your care partners to advocate for themselves and remain active and engaged in their healthcare will assist in preserving their dignity and ultimately, combat ageism and any other form of discrimination they may face.

In Table 4.1, I summarize key strategies and provide examples of how, through communication with patients and healthcare providers, you can work to combat ageism.

Table 4.1: Communication Strategies to Help Combat Ageism

Strategy	Sample questions to implement the strategy
Explore beliefs you and your care partner have about their age and the impact of their age on the type of care that should be received.	**Ask yourself:** • Do I feel like my care partner is too old to receive [insert medical procedure, device, etc.]? Why or why not? • In what ways is their age impacting the decisions we are jointly making about their healthcare? **Ask your care partner:** • Do you feel like you are too old to receive [insert medical procedure, device, etc.]? Why or why not? • In what ways is your age impacting the decisions you are making about your healthcare? • If you were younger, would you feel differently about the treatment you're receiving? Why or why not?

Strategy	Sample questions to implement the strategy
Address elderspeak and other verbal and nonverbal discriminatory behaviors when communicating with healthcare professionals.	**Ask the healthcare professional:** • Can you please speak to him slower and with a lower tone so that he can understand you better? • Would it be possible for you to sit next to his bed so that he can see your face more clearly when you speak? • Can you please speak to him directly? • Can you please refer to him by his name?
Ask clarifying questions if you or your care partner do not understand what the healthcare professional is saying.	**Ask your care partner:** • Did you understand what [insert name of healthcare professional] just said? **Ask the healthcare professional:** • [Insert name of healthcare professional], can you please explain a bit more about what you mean by that? • What does [insert medical term] mean?
Ask your care partner to summarize what the conversation was about, and what if anything was decided about the medical plan moving forward.	**Ask your care partner:** • Can you summarize what [insert name of healthcare professional] just said? What do you understand to be the options moving forward?

Caregivers Are Vulnerable to Discrimination, Too

Ageism can happen at any age, and as a caregiver, you are not immune to it or to any other form of discrimination. According to the National Alliance for Caregiving, of the over 53 million American caregivers, 17 percent identify as Hispanic/Latino, 14 percent identify as African American, 8 percent identify as a sexual and gender minority (SGM), and 5 percent identify as Asian American or Pacific Islander.[34] One out of every four American Indian and Alaska Native adults identify themselves as a family caregiver.[35] As these numbers are anticipated to grow in the coming years, the aggregate number of family caregivers from diverse communities will outnumber non-Hispanic White and non-SGM caregivers.[36] This means that an increasing number of you may be faced with discrimination or bias of some kind as a caregiver, such as healthcare professionals assuming you don't understand English, healthcare professionals assuming that you will not understand complex information and providing you with only the bare minimum, and healthcare professionals not taking you seriously if you are younger, male, or disabled.[37]

During many of our ER visits, it seemed like my dad and I represented the youngest and oldest partners in care; our sixty-year age difference was always an element of our story, and I often wondered if being a young woman impacted the way healthcare professionals interacted with me and, by extension, my dad. I often found myself hypothesizing that if I were older, or male, I might be treated differently by some of the staff. In fact, regardless of which hospital my dad was brought to by ambulance, I would put on my hospital identification badge to buffer the personal sense of authority I felt was sometimes questioned just by looking at me. I felt like I, too, needed to tell my story in some way to help ensure the best possible outcome for my dad. I frequently shared, almost defensively, that I was a psychologist and that I specialized in supporting families of patients with cancer. I wanted to be taken seriously by all those caring for my dad, and to prophylactically combat any assumptions about who I was (the uninformed daughter? the demanding daughter?).

Now that I am no longer in the thick of the intensity of these moments, I can see clearly how my burnout made me more sensitive when communicating with healthcare professionals. Each time a member of the medical team would speak to me without making eye contact contributed to my feelings of invisibility. Each time a belittling tone was used, I found myself questioning what it was that I was saying. It would have been so much more powerful and effective for those healthcare professionals to interact with me in a more engaged manner, as if I was a peer, an ad hoc member of the healthcare team. What I did in those moments—and what I encourage you to do—is I modeled the way I *wanted to be spoken to as a caregiver* by how I spoke to them in return. When I responded, I made a point to maintain eye contact, I used a steady and calm tone of voice, and I asked clarifying questions so that I could have my concerns addressed.

While I had certainly experienced interactions with healthcare team members that were blatantly disrespectful of me, my sheer exhaustion made me sensitive in almost all conversations. As a result, I frequently became the victim of my own unhelpful thinking. I found myself engaging in mind reading and overgeneralization, two of the thought patterns I highlighted in Chapter 3. One form of mind reading is assuming that someone is reacting negatively to you without evidence to support this fact. This can result in misinterpreting facial expressions or tones of voice in a negative way, something I frequently found myself doing when speaking with members of the medical team. The striking, difficult interactions with healthcare professionals I had early on in 2013 led me to overgeneralize and assume that I would have similar experiences moving forward. In effect, through mind reading and overgeneralization, I allowed those early negative experiences with healthcare professionals to shape the way that I interpreted most subsequent interactions.

Looking back, I wish I had engaged in cognitive restructuring in those moments to combat my unhelpful thinking and to recognize the role I was playing in making those moments more difficult for myself. Undoubtedly, as I stood by my dad, I was the expert and I understood him better than any of his providers ever could have. This is what I want you to hold on to. It is critical that you internalize the fact that *you* are an authority on your loved one's care, you have a better understanding of their day-to-day functioning than any healthcare professional could ever have, and your voice and perspective is necessary for your loved one to receive the care they deserve.

Early on in my faculty role at Memorial Sloan Kettering Cancer Center, a handful of patients said some version of "You're Dr. Applebaum? I expected someone more experienced" when they would meet me for the first time in the Counseling Center waiting room. In those interactions, it felt like my age was associated with a judgment about my capacity to provide high-quality psychosocial care. While I took (silent) offense in those moments, during the same period I remember meeting a young-appearing neurologist who was taking care of my dad when he was in the coma and *having the exact same thought*; I assumed that an older physician would have been able to provide my dad with a higher level of care. I was guilty of the exact same bias of which I was also the victim! It was only through examining my own assumptions about age and competence that I was able to work against my own ageist beliefs.

In addition to addressing ways in which you and your care partner are the recipients of discrimination, I encourage you to reflect on any ways your own behaviors, beliefs, and identities might reveal potential biases and assumptions about your loved one's care team, whether they fall into the category of ageism or any other type of discrimination.

* * *

I remember the feeling I had when I took my dad for his first appointment with a new internist who had come highly recommended as someone who specialized in working with older adults. It was in 2014 after my dad's intense year of hospitalizations and nursing home stays. He was in a wheelchair, and I accompanied him and the home health aide. The doctor conducted a comprehensive interview, as most physicians do with new patients coming in for a physical, but what stood out to me were the types of questions he asked: "What is a typical day like for you, Stan?" "What brings you enjoyment these days?" "How do your feet feel?" These and many, many others were questions I don't ever remember being asked of my dad in other settings. They were questions that addressed the lived reality of being Stanley Applebaum in his nineties.

In that first meeting, in addition to hearing about my dad's medical history and the current challenges he was having physically, that doctor truly got to know my dad. For example, he learned of my dad's lifelong drive to respond to limitations as opportunities for learning. My dad shared that as a child he was frail and suffered from pleurisy and was told that his heart was weak, and that as a result, his initial dreams included wanting to be a physician so that he could solve the medical problems with which he had been faced. With a few more questions, that doctor learned of my dad's ingenuity in the face of challenges, and how he was able to use his musical talents to save his life when he served in the United States Army in World War II. When the war in Europe ended, his battalion was in Wiesbaden, Germany, and he convinced the commanding officer that he could use his pianist fingers to work as a teletypist and convey important communications to Washington. As a result, he was transferred to the Special Services and avoided traveling to fight in Japan, eventually making it back safely home. Turning to the present time, that doctor subsequently learned how important it was for my dad to continue to make the most of each day, to feel productive in some way, and to continue to enjoy life through his five senses despite his physical limitations. This meant spending time each week working with my mom at the piano before her death; being able to continue to create music and children's stories and poetry; engaging in meaningful conversations with me and my brother and his friends from the music industry; having a drink occasionally of champagne; listening to music; getting lost in laughter; and connecting to love through tight hand-holds and hugs. The questions that doctor asked weren't pathologizing; they didn't focus on his Lewy body disease but on what living life fully at that time meant to my dad. In that room, I took an exhale. I felt validated and held. As did my dad, who after the appointment looked at me with the biggest smile and told me how much he liked that doctor and then asked if we could finally make that appointment with the podiatrist we had been putting off for months.

While there is rarely time for these types of conversations when you accompany your care partner in the ER, they should be integrated into discussions with primary care physicians and specialists regularly involved in their outpatient care. If the healthcare team taking care of your loved one is not asking these types of questions organically, take a few minutes to start these conversations yourself. It will allow everyone involved to make valuable connections that can have significant downstream effects on the care that is delivered.

Functional versus Chronological Age

What that doctor was doing was assessing my dad's functional age. Chronological age alone is generally a poor indicator of the physiological and functional status of older adults. Aging is a heterogeneous process, which means that two ninety-year-olds can have vastly different physical, cognitive, and emotional abilities. Functional age takes into consideration these differences and addresses the overall functioning of an individual and accounts for genetics, lifestyle, nutrition, and other diseases and conditions. It also reflects the cumulative effects of both medical and psychosocial stressors—caregiving responsibilities included—on aging. Functional age is therefore more comprehensive and meaningful than what can be conveyed by a date of birth on a hospital wristband.

The benefits of conducting assessments of functional age among older adults are profound. My dad was, chronologically, in his early nineties before he was diagnosed with Lewy body disease or faced any significant physical challenges and at that point, his functional age was much different than his date of birth suggested. And so, when he became ill and was hospitalized, what I was doing each time I stood by as the rounding team examined my dad was advocating for his functional age. I was striving for the medical team members to replace an image of a frail ninety-something-year-old nuanced with assumptions and biases with the full range of human potential that existed in the individual in the bed in front of them. This, then, is your job as a caregiver—to convey your loved one's functional age so that they may receive the most comprehensive care possible.

Many of the questions my dad's doctor asked that day were similar to those that are part of a more formal geriatric assessment, which can be used to provide a comprehensive overview of an older adult's functional abilities, physical performance, nutritional status, comorbidities, cognition, psychological state, and social support system.[38] This type of assessment provides much more meaningful and personalized data than chronological age in isolation. The most informative assessments include an evaluation of older adults' capacities to engage in activities of daily living and instrumental activities of daily living, as well as objective measures of physical functioning, such as their ability to walk independently, balance, grip strength, leg strength, and history of falls.[39] In addition to interviewing my dad and eventually learning of his experiences in World War II and his career in music, that doctor also directed several questions at me and the aide to learn more about my dad's day-to-day functioning and healthcare needs. Our subsequent visits were all equally comprehensive, caring, and attentive; he never once appeared to treat my dad differently because of his age. He spoke to him in the same tone as he did with me and the aide, made a point to sit so that he and my dad were on equal ground and eye level when communicating, and advocated for interventions that would allow my dad to live as long as possible, outside the hospital, with the best quality of life.

The goal of a geriatric assessment is to guide treatment planning and provide potential interventions to improve the general health and quality of life of older people. Such evaluations can lead to the provision of personalized care, that is, care that is appropriate based on the patient's unique needs. For my dad, this included taking steps to honor his goal of staying out of the hospital except in life-or-death circumstances through enrolling him in a visiting doctor's program, and promoting his quality of life through a prescription for new hearing aids and occupational therapy. Geriatric assessments should be comprehensive and include an evaluation of the following: all existing medical conditions; cognition, including cognitive impairment, dementia, and history of delirium; medication use, including psychiatric medications; existing social support; and social functioning, psychological well-being, and nutritional status.[40] Perhaps not surprisingly, among older adults being treated for cancer who receive geriatric assessments, studies have shown that treatment plans are modified in more than a third of patients after the evaluation to reflect patients' goals for promoting quality of life.[41]

While geriatric assessments should undoubtedly become a standard of care in the treatment of older adults, as of today they are not consistently implemented. If this is the case in the setting where your loved one is receiving care, I encourage you to reflect on the domains of functioning listed in Table 4.2 and to address them with your care partner's healthcare providers. I've included suggested action items and discussion points that can help you to promote the independence and quality of life of your loved one, for as long as possible, through focusing on each of these domains of functioning.

Table 4.2: Assessment Domains for Older Adults to Promote Quality of Life

Domain	Example	Caregiver To-Do
Activities of daily living	Independence in bathing, grooming, feeding, toileting, dressing, walking.	If your care partner is unable to perform these tasks independently, what support can be implemented at home? What changes can be made to ensure safety at home? Examples include the installation of grab bars and shower chairs to make bathing safer, and the removal of rugs to help prevent tripping and falling.
Instrumental activities of daily living	Independence in meal preparation, shopping, housework, managing finances, transportation, using technology.	What tasks are most important to your care partner to do on their own? What can be delegated and to whom? If your care partner has difficulty using technology such as smartphones, can you buy them an adaptive phone with a larger screen and keys? What other steps can you take to promote your care partner's capacity to carry out these tasks independently?
Cognition	Memory, attention, concentration.	What aids can be used to help your care partner cope with limitations? Tools such as pill boxes labeled with the days of the week and Post-it notes around the house can be helpful.

Domain	Example	Caregiver To-Do
Social support	Availability of emotional, informational, tangible, affectionate, and positive social interaction.	Does your care partner feel well supported? Are there individuals—outside of yourself—who provide them with consistent support? Are there community-based organizations, religious communities, and other programs that can serve as additional sources of support?
Emotional status	Presence of emotional concerns, such as anxiety, depression, and insomnia.	Does your care partner feel comfortable discussing their emotional health with you? If not, do they have a trusted friend to confide in? Does your care partner receive support from a mental health professional? If not, would they be willing to receive professional support?
Nutrition status	Significant weight gain or weight loss in the past six months.	Does your care partner cook for themselves? Would assistance with food shopping and meal preparation help to address nutritional concerns? Consult with a nutritionist about dietary changes that can assist with maintaining a healthy weight if you haven't already. This person can usually be recommended by a primary care physician.

Domain	Example	Caregiver To-Do
Hearing	Hearing quality, use of hearing aids, effectiveness of hearing aids.	If your care partner has difficulty hearing, taking steps to secure hearing aids can have a tremendous positive impact on their quality of life.
Vision	Vision quality, wearing glasses/contacts, effectiveness of glasses/contacts.	Does your care partner need an eye exam? When is the last time their prescription was updated? Even subtle problems with vision can have a significant and negative impact on quality of life.
Life Goals*	Specific to each individual, these can include the desire to continue working, to be present for specific events, to travel, to engage in meaningful activities.	**Ask your care partner:** • What are you not doing that you wish you were doing? What brings you the most joy? • How can I/we help you to do more of that? • What does meaningful life look like to you right now?

Each of these domains is a critical aspect of functioning that should be assessed and taken into consideration when you, your care partner, and the medical team are coming up with a plan of care. Assessing them will also allow for the implementation of often simple but powerful interventions when available (for example, prescriptions for glasses and/or hearing aids), which can have a dramatic impact on your loved one's quality of life and facilitate their engage-

---

* Life Goals is not a traditional category on geriatric assessments, but I strongly believe that it should be.

ment in healthcare communication and, more importantly, life in general. While the last domain in Table 4.2 is not integrated into most existing assessments, I strongly believe goals of life should be included as well. Just as discussing goals of care (the topic of the next chapter) is critical in assisting patients to receive value-driven care, so too is assessment and discussion of goals of life, especially in the context of working against ageism. Exploring these goals will help you to take steps to maximize your care partner's quality of life, and the quality of the time you have together.

These goals of life were a regular part of my conversations with my dad. In fact, an enduring theme of our father-daughter dialogue was how we could each uniquely and together make the most of every day. Once my dad was bedbound, these discussions focused on how, in the face of his limitations, he could continue to choose to live each day to its fullest. These limitations included severely compromised vision, which due to Lewy body disease could not be corrected with glasses, and tremulous hands, both of which challenged his ability to play the piano and hold the small silver pencil and ruler that had accompanied him for nearly seventy-five years as he wrote music. So instead of writing music the old-fashioned way, he would spend hours thinking about musical arrangements he had done in the past and would reconfigure them to come up with an entirely new take on the piece. He was able to document his new ideas in voice memos that I or the home health aides recorded on our phones, or on a few occasions, musician friends of mine joined him to take down on paper what he was orchestrating in his mind. These experiences allowed him to remain connected to the musician in him who was such a driver of who he had been for his entire life. He similarly spent time on most days writing children's stories and poetry, which he dictated to the home health aides and which I eventually typed up.

My dad was a lifelong learner, and meaningful life meant continuing to learn and grow, despite his limitations. In addition to asking his home health aides to teach him Tagalog, every week I would print out articles from the Science section of the *New York Times* in large font and put Scotch tape on the edge of the pages. This accommodated his limited vision and compromised sensation in his fingertips and allowed him to hold and turn the pages at his own pace. Inevitably, each article would turn into a million questions about topics ranging from quantum physics to global warming and inspired within him the desire to read and learn more.

After my mom's death, my dad and I created a New Year's Eve tradition to help him cope with the loss of nearly forty-five years of celebrating with her: We would each write our goals for the next year on little pieces of paper and put them into mini champagne bottles which we had emptied into the finest crystal to enjoy for a toast. These annual goals eventually made it into the conversations we had with my dad's doctors to help us frame his goals for life, and by extension, his goals for care. Just as it was important for me and my dad to discuss them, it was necessary for his doctors to understand what he wanted to get out of life, so that steps could be taken to ensure the greatest chance of those goals being met.

I encourage you to engage in your own version of this exercise so that your care partner's life goals can be clearly communicated to members of the healthcare team. In many ways, doing so is a powerful way to combat ageism. Advocating for your care partner to live life as fully as possible—whatever that uniquely means to them—for as long as possible, will help to ensure that age-related biases are not shaping the treatment they receive.

On December 31, 2018, we completed our tradition one last time. My dad's goals for the coming year were not about *doing* life but instead about *receiving* life. He wanted to spend time outside in the sunshine. He wanted to sip Stewart's root beer and eat ice cream. He wanted to hold my first book. He wanted to meet his second grandson. He wanted to experience as much love as possible despite his limited energy. His goals for life that year were no less meaningful or important or valid than those he shared in 2014. During the seven weeks of 2019 that he lived, all of his goals were met. I focused during that time on doing everything I could to ensure that the ways that my dad received life through his five senses, through the experiences of love, and beauty, and humor, were as complete and rich and fulfilling as possible.

As his goals changed, so too did mine. And so will yours. Inevitably, our goals of life as caregivers are intimately tied to our care partner's goals of life. While it can be painful to witness shifting goals, helping to ensure that your loved one's goals of life are achieved is one of the greatest gifts that you can give them, and ultimately, will become one of the greatest gifts you can give yourself.

CHAPTER 5

Care Is Not One-Size-Fits-All

Save the Last Dance for Me

Artist: Ben E. King and The Drifters
Arranged and Conducted by Stan Applebaum, 1960

Discussions about advance care planning are often among the most important—and most difficult—you will have as caregivers, and you are uniquely positioned to guide them. Caregivers frequently have a more accurate understanding of patients' prognoses than patients themselves[1] and are increasingly relied on to manage a range of demanding responsibilities in decision-making.[2] Optimal outcomes, including your ability to carry out your loved one's goals of care, therefore, may hinge on your ability to initiate and navigate these complex yet necessary discussions. These discussions impact not only the care your loved one receives and their quality of life but your experience during caregiving and beyond as well. In this chapter, I provide an overview of the main facets of advance care planning and specific skills and tools that you can use to facilitate these discussions with your care partner and members of the healthcare team. Although challenging, these conversations are important opportunities to connect more deeply with your loved one and when engaged with courage and vulnerability, can allow you to feel more in control of your caregiving journey.

✽   ✽   ✽

From the very first hospitalization until my dad's last weeks of life, I was asked by medical professionals at all ranks of the hospital hierarchy about his goals of care. *Goals of care* include the goals patients have for the care they are currently receiving, as well as care they will receive in the near future and over the long term. Goals of care include what patients value in terms of their desire to receive care that can save or extend their lives, as well as care that is focused primarily on preserving their quality of life, however long that may be. These goals of care inform treatment choices, such as patients being willing to receive cardiopulmonary resuscitation (CPR) if a cardiac arrest were to occur, or for patients with cancer, receiving chemotherapy that would lead to some chance of a cure but that could come with a high side effect profile, versus care that is palliative and focused primarily on addressing symptoms and quality of life. Importantly, goals of care are not static. Instead, in most cases, they shift over the course of an illness trajectory and more broadly, one's life.

I repeat: *goals of care are not static.*

My dad and I spoke openly and repeatedly about treatment goals throughout our time as partners in care, and I made a commitment to carrying those out until he took his last breath. My dad's goals of care had emerged from the repeated discussions we had about advance care planning. *Advance care planning* is an umbrella term for the process of thinking ahead to goals of care, treatment choices, and choosing a healthcare proxy to speak for oneself at a point in the future. Advance care planning includes the completion of advanced directives, legal documents that outline our goals of care and how—ideally—we would like them to be carried out.

My first conversation with my dad about advance care planning occurred on the drive to school in October 1999. I was seventeen; my dad was seventy-seven. My maternal grandmother had just died, and we had returned the day before from her funeral in Pittsburgh. I asked him about the customs I had just witnessed, and eventually got the courage to ask him if that's how he envisioned his funeral, and if he had any thoughts on how he would like to die. "In my sleep," he said. "And a pine box is fine, just make sure you find the least expensive one. It's just going to disintegrate." Always concerned about finances, he then turned the conversation to the extraordinary racket that is the business side of dying.

Eleven years later he and I broached the topic again when he was being discharged after a hospitalization for a cellulitis infection. This was shortly after I finished graduate school and moved back to New York. I asked what his goals were at that time, and if he got sick again, if he would want to go back to the hospital and receive the type of lifesaving care that he just had. He answered in the affirmative but felt strongly that he wouldn't want to be kept alive by machines. Nonetheless, these answers were accompanied by qualifications. "I'm not ready to go; there is life to be lived," he said.

We revisited these topics when I formally became my dad's healthcare proxy after my mom's death in 2014. He once again shared that he was not ready to die and would want to be taken to the hospital if he got sick. He also chose not to sign a Do-Not-Resuscitate (DNR) order. He and I had spoken at length about the meaning of this form—not just what was stated on the paper but also the implications of signing on the care and attention he might receive in the hospital. We spoke about how, during the prior fifteen months in which he had eight hospitalizations and seven stays in nursing facilities and spent one month in a coma, had he signed a DNR order, it was unlikely that he would be sitting with me having that discussion. He understood that the actions of the medical team were dictated in many ways by DNR status, and he wondered if, for example, on the occasions when he appeared to be becoming septic because of urinary tract infections, he would have received the same urgent care in the hospital had he signed the DNR order. Importantly, we discussed how this was a conversation and a decision he could return to, and I knew that he would make his wishes clear to me if they changed.

The Importance of Repeated Conversations

What I was doing with my dad, and what I encourage you to do, was repeatedly opening conversations about advance care planning. This is not a conversation that should happen only once. Certainly, it is anxiety provoking and scary to open these discussions, but like any difficult conversation, they get easier with each repetition. Repetition is important because as patients move through their illness journeys, what they envision as appropriate care often changes. For sure, the decisions we made on behalf of my dad in 2013 were different than those made in 2019; I knew from repeated conversations that his goals of care had changed. Therefore, it will be important for you to engage in *open* and *honest* and *repeated* conversations with your loved ones about their goals of care, their values, and what matters to them at the end of life so that you can feel confident that you can carry forward their goals.

Even though my dad and I had these repeated conversations, each time I felt the need to call an ambulance to get him to the hospital, if it was not a moment of absolute crisis and he was awake enough to engage, I asked him for permission to call that ambulance. I wanted to confirm that we remained on the same page. On the occasions when he was unable to engage in these discussions, I never once questioned my decision to take him to the hospital because I knew from our repeated conversations that he felt that there was more meaningful life to be lived and he was not ready to "leave" (his phrase). The confidence I felt in decision-making after having had these conversations is confidence that I hope you, too, will feel.

Most of you who identify as the primary caregiver for a patient will likely be designated as their healthcare proxy, though of course there are exceptions to this. Serving as a healthcare proxy is a significant responsibility, and while proxy forms are often addressed for the first time when patients are admitted to the hospital for acute care, the magnitude of the responsibility is often realized long after those events. As a healthcare proxy, you will have the same rights to request or refuse treatment that your loved ones would have if they could make and communicate decisions. While the designation of a healthcare proxy involves the completion of a legal document, your role and responsibilities are much more significant than a piece of paper. The most important function of this role is assumed if there is a point at which your care partner is no longer able to make healthcare decisions for themself, when they don't "have capacity." This can happen when, for whatever reason, they are not conscious or able to communicate on their own behalf. In those moments, for you to carry out their goals of care, it will be necessary for you to be aware of these goals, in advance of that moment.

Many caregivers have shared with me how scared they are of making the "wrong" decisions as healthcare proxies. Is this something you have felt? This feeling is normal, and it's certainly something both my mom and I experienced when we were faced with making decisions on my dad's behalf. When he was in the coma in 2013 and my mom was his designated healthcare proxy, she was asked whether the medical team could perform a lumbar puncture that might help to determine an appropriate plan of care. That day, we discussed what my dad would say if he were able to speak on his own behalf, and it became clear that he would want at least a chance of treatment and meaningful survival, if one could be determined by the procedure. My mom's consenting to the lumbar puncture was her way of bringing my dad's voice into the room. Like every caregiver, I've certainly second-guessed myself while reflecting back across the years that I advocated for my dad's goals of care. However, I'm reminded that the decisions my mom and I made weren't our decisions. They were my dad's decisions. Similarly, the decisions you will make will not be yours. They will be your care partner's decisions, and your responsibility in those situations is to represent those wishes as best you can.

Not surprisingly, discussions about advance care planning can be emotionally challenging, and many caregivers feel unprepared to have these conversations in the first place. So it is completely normal and appropriate for you to feel fearful of beginning them as well. My guess is that just reading the first few pages of this chapter and imagining opening these discussions might be anxiety provoking. (If so, this is a great moment to put into practice that diaphragmatic breathing technique I included at the end of Chapter 3.) Moreover, while you might be ready and willing to have these conversations, their success depends equally on you *and* your partner in care, who may not be nearly as ready as you to discuss the future. Remember this if you are met with resistance when you open these discussions. Additionally, long-standing communication patterns, including avoidant coping styles in which difficult topics are shoved under the rug, can make opening these conversations in the present moment even more difficult. It takes courage to begin these discussions, and even if you feel like you haven't accomplished them fully, I hope you will feel proud of yourself for trying.

Like many caregivers, Carol was fearful of bringing up the topic of advance care planning. She was a thirty-five-year-old teacher in the New York City public school system and came to see me soon after her husband, Ethan, forty-one, was diagnosed with advanced colorectal cancer. Ethan's cancer had been discovered after he suffered for several months with gastrointestinal distress that had been previously dismissed as "stress-related," symptoms that came on several grueling months after he began working as a police officer with the New York Police Department. He eventually went to his primary care doctor, who recommended a colonoscopy that revealed a large mass on his colon. A subsequent MRI indicated that the cancer had spread to Ethan's liver. Soon after receiving this news, he underwent surgery and began an aggressive form of chemotherapy that his oncologist said would be difficult to tolerate but would give him the best chance of surviving and even thriving post cancer.

Our first session occurred after Ethan's surgery, soon after he began chemotherapy. Carol shared how traumatic the diagnosis experience was for them, how sad it was for her to see Ethan suffering the side effects of chemotherapy, and how challenging it was for her to cope with intensifying worry about Ethan's survival. The couple had married just a year earlier and were beginning to plan for starting a family right around the time of the diagnosis. Cancer was completely unexpected. In those first few sessions, much of the focus was on how desperately Carol wanted to speak to Ethan about the future, about scenarios in which the treatment stopped working. Carol had no sense of what type of care Ethan would want in the future, the extent to which prolonging life versus promoting quality of life was important to him, or whether Ethan would want to sign a Do-Not-Resuscitate (DNR) or Do-Not-Intubate (DNI) order. Carol shared her fear that if she were to bring up these topics with Ethan, it would cause extraordinary distress that would then have a negative impact on his recovery. She told me that up until our first session, she had spent energy actively hiding her fears and trying to maintain an optimistic and hopeful tone in all her conversations with Ethan.

I suggested to Carol that it was very likely that she and Ethan were in a cycle that I call a *network of silence,* what my colleague Dr. Andrew Roth calls *the tension of good intentions:*[3] The worries she was having were likely worries that Ethan, too, was having, and it was possible that Ethan was also holding back from discussing these topics out of fear of upsetting Carol. While emerging from good intentions, networks of silence prevent you from discussing what is most important, from disclosing worries and concerns that are likely shared by your loved one. Such withholding creates feelings of isolation and alienation. Certainly, opening up can be difficult, but doing so allows partners in care to support one another. Again and again, I've seen these conversations engender greater emotional vulnerability and closeness.

I encouraged Carol to write out a list of all the questions and topics that she wanted to discuss with Ethan so that she could have them clearly outlined in front of her. I described the benefits of starting this conversation by setting an agenda and summarizing what Carol wanted to talk about and why, and asking Ethan if there was anything he wanted to add to this list. I then encouraged her to pick a time to open the conversation, which I emphasized would likely be repeated. We discussed the importance of timing these conversations for when they could both give their full attention and focus, so Carol decided to start this conversation on a Saturday morning when Ethan was off from work. We also discussed the benefits of planning for something pleasurable the two could do after, such as a walk through the botanical gardens together.

When Carol returned the following week, she shared how pleasantly surprised she was by how well the conversation went. Ethan was willing to schedule a time to have this discussion, and he agreed that talking through Carol's official role as healthcare proxy was important. Ethan expressed feeling intensely guilty about getting sick and the burden he felt he was placing on Carol's shoulders. He described wanting to protect Carol and his fear of what his illness might do to her emotionally. He also disclosed that he had no idea what type of care he would want in the future and that thinking about the future was overwhelming to him. As a result of this discussion, Carol felt ready to sign a healthcare proxy form and more comfortable with repeating the conversation in the future. And for Ethan, the discussion highlighted how distressed he was and how beneficial it would be for him, too, to be in therapy.

Fast forward to three years later. After more than a year of Ethan's cancer being in remission, it recurred. Carol was devastated. She saw Ethan change physically and noticed that the hardiness he exhibited during his first round of treatment was no longer present. However, since we had first met, Carol and Ethan had continued to speak openly about what Ethan valued in terms of his life, and his care; their Saturday morning conversations had morphed into a regular part of their routine. He made it clear to Carol that he wanted to live as long as possible, but that living meant being able to be active and engaged socially, to be able to enjoy life. He shared that if there was a time when he could no longer engage meaningfully in life, and if his symptoms were severe and debilitating, that type of life wouldn't be life worth living. Despite Ethan's worsening health, Carol felt more confident in her ability to support and advocate for him, and more capable of being fully present and enjoying each moment with him to its fullest.

When Carol returned to see me for support shortly before Ethan transitioned to hospice care, she shared that despite the intense sadness she felt—her anticipatory grief was strong—she was confident that she knew what Ethan wanted and could carry out his wishes if necessary. Ethan ultimately signed DNR and DNI orders, and clearly expressed that his wishes included being lucid and awake for as long as possible, which meant potentially limiting the use of pain medications until absolutely necessary. Having both engaged in psychotherapy, Carol and Ethan realized the benefit of support and enlisted the help of a death doula, an individual who supported the couple during Ethan's last days, and who continued to provide support to Carol in bereavement.

Despite how scary these initial conversations were, the courage Carol demonstrated in opening them paid off: She set the stage for an incredibly honest dialogue about what meaningful life meant and ways in which she and Ethan could support each other. After Ethan's death, Carol shared that these conversations had engendered a deepening of love between them and greater respect for one other. She also told me that she felt proud of herself for the courage she had shown during his illness and in how she was able to honor his wishes. This pride ultimately contributed to her moving through her grief without significant mental health concerns.

How to Have the Tough Conversations

As with Carol, there are strategies you can use to facilitate conversations with your loved ones and members of the healthcare team about advance care planning. Many of these strategies have been tested and subsequently taught as part of a communication skills training program developed at Memorial Sloan Kettering Cancer Center.[4] In Table 5.1, I've provided an overview of these strategies and examples of things you can do to move toward achieving your advance care planning communication goals.

Table 5.1: Strategies to Facilitate Advance Care Planning Discussions

Strategy	Examples	Helpful Tips
Agenda setting	−Declare agenda items −Provide rationale for the conversation −Negotiate agenda, if necessary	−Acknowledge the importance of discussing advance care planning in helping you to carry out your caregiving responsibilities −Invite your care partner to add to the agenda **For example:** • I would really like to talk about where you would like to receive care at the end of your life so that I can do everything possible to make sure your wishes are honored. Is that okay? Is there anything you'd like to speak with me about?
Work toward a shared understanding of your care partner's goals of care	−Ask open-ended questions −Clarify information shared −Restate to assure understanding −Summarize information shared −Encourage expression of feelings	−Validate the emotional intensity of the topic **Ask questions like:** • What matters to you at the end of life? • When you think about the last phase of your life, what's most important to you in terms of the care you receive? • Who would you prefer to be involved in decisions about your care? • What would you consider to be a good or meaningful death?

Empathically respond to your care partner's emotion	—Acknowledge —Validate —Normalize	—Use silence to provide space for your loved one to express their emotions —Validate the emotional intensity of the topic **For example:** • I know this is painful to talk about. It's hard for me, too.
Discuss goals for the upcoming visit with the health-care professional (i.e., "consent conversation")	—Provide a rationale for the conversation —Restate to assure understanding —Summarize information shared —Encourage expression of feelings	—Validate the emotional intensity of the topic **Ask questions like:** • Are you comfortable with our discussing your prognosis with Dr. X? • Are there any topics that you do not want to discuss with Dr. X?
When meeting with the health-care professional, work toward a shared under-standing of your care partner's prognosis	—Ask open-ended questions —Clarify information shared —Restate to assure understanding	—Ask for a moment to gather thoughts **Ask questions like:** • What can we expect his quality of life to be like in the future? • Could the tumor be gone forever, or should we expect it to eventually come back?
Discuss goals of care in a straight-forward manner with the health-care professional	—Clarify information shared —Restate to assure understanding	—Facilitate a dialogue be-tween yourself, your loved one, and the healthcare professional **Ask questions like:** • Would it be possible to talk about what steps are available to take if this treatment stops working?

All the strategies listed in Table 5.1 are helpful in achieving communication goals, but I want to highlight two that are particularly powerful in helping you to navigate these difficult discussions. The first is agenda setting, which involves sharing an agenda for the conversation you want to have with your care partner (such as "I would really like for us to talk about . . ."), providing a rationale for the conversation (for example, ". . . because it's important that I understand what type of care you want"), and asking your care partner if there is anything they would like to add to the agenda ("If there are other topics you'd like to discuss, we can make sure to get to them, too"). Since opening conversations about advance care planning can be anxiety-provoking, having a plan for how to begin these discussions can be incredibly helpful; setting the agenda allows you to make your intentions clear. Additionally, many caregivers have found that practicing setting the agenda in advance of the actual conversation, such as with a trusted friend, helps them to feel more confident when they do so with their loved one.

The second strategy I want to highlight is the consent conversation. Many caregivers have told me that when they accompany their care partners to doctors' appointments, they often want to ask certain questions but are afraid to do so for fear of upsetting them. While intended to minimize anxiety and distress, this holding back from discussing certain topics—this *network of silence*, this *tension of good intentions*—eventually has the opposite effect for many families who are desperate to have open conversations with members of the healthcare team about the future. To address this, I encourage you to have the consent conversation long in advance of the next visit with the doctor. At the heart of this conversation is your stating what it is you would like to speak about in the next visit with the doctor, and checking in to see if your loved one is okay with your discussing that topic. For example, you could say, "I would really love for us to talk with your doctor about what treatment options are available if this current treatment stops working. Would that be okay?" As with setting the agenda, when engaging in a consent conversation, providing a rationale for the discussion and encouraging your loved one to add to the topics to be covered is important. Moreover, to ensure that you both are on the same page, it's helpful for you to summarize what was discussed and to restate your understanding to ensure that you both will be comfortable in the upcoming visit. For example, you might say something like, "It sounds like you're okay with my asking your doctor about what other treatment options are available, but not the chances of this current treatment working. Is that correct?" Importantly, if your loved one is not comfortable with discussing certain topics, it can be beneficial to validate those feelings by saying something like, "It's fine if you don't want to discuss that topic during tomorrow's visit. Would it be okay if I ask you again in a few months when we have our next appointment with the doctor?" In Table 5.1, I've listed additional questions that you can use to facilitate these discussions.

These are not easy conversations to have, even for the most seasoned conversationalists. Be mindful of having them at a time when everyone has the emotional space to explore their thoughts. Let the strategies outlined in Table 5.1 assist you in preparing for and opening these discussions. Finally, it's important that you allow yourself to express the range of difficult emotions that might be triggered along the way. It can also be helpful to schedule something pleasurable after these conversations—such as a coffee date with a trusted friend—to ensure that social support is available and emotional expression is supported.

Despite how challenging they can be, these conversations are worth it; discussions about advance care planning can have a positive impact on many critical outcomes, including what you and your loved ones understand about their illness and what to expect in terms of how the illness will respond to certain treatments, and your—and your care partner's—mental health.[5] Such conversations are also great opportunities to ensure that you and your care partner understand what is meant by the terms *palliative care* and *hospice care*, which too often get confused with one another.

Palliative care refers to medical care that focuses on improving quality of life by managing symptoms associated with serious illness, such as pain and fatigue. While palliative care services are often offered to patients with life-limiting illnesses toward the end of life, the benefits of palliative care for patients and caregivers early on in illness journeys are significant.[6] Importantly, palliative care involves mental health care, including mental health care for caregivers such as yourselves.

Hospice care, on the other hand, refers to services that focus on the care, comfort, and quality of life of patients who are approaching the end of life to promote quality of life *and* death. Hospice services can be delivered at home or in an inpatient facility, and while they include palliative care, palliative care does not by definition include hospice care. This distinction is important, as many caregivers are fearful of speaking with members of the palliative care team and assume that doing so will mean the death of their care partner is imminent. Discussing the meaning of these terms with your care partner and learning about what matters to them at the end of life is a critical component of advance care planning.

According to the Institute of Medicine, a "good death" is free from avoidable distress and suffering for patients and families; is in accord with patients' and families' wishes; and is consistent with clinical, cultural, and ethical standards.[7] In clinic, I've often asked patients and caregivers, "What would you consider to be a good or meaningful death?" a question drawn from an approach I discuss in Chapter 9. From patients' perspectives, answers usually include a death experience that involves limited physical pain and suffering and that allows patients some element of control. Such experiences are often achieved with the help of a hospice team in place. Importantly, while we may not have control over how we ultimately die, we often can decide where we would like to die and, among other things, in whose company.

For caregivers who reflect on what a "good death" would be for their loved ones, answers are often similarly focused on deaths that are as free as possible of suffering. Caregivers frequently share with me that a priority for them is that their loved one's death occurs in a manner that is in line with their loved one's wishes. In bereavement, being able to reflect on the patient's death and know that it occurred in a manner that honored these wishes has significant mental health benefits,[8] as was the case for Carol. Conversely, the post-traumatic stress symptomatology I see in bereaved caregivers frequently results from not being able to carry out a loved one's wishes at the end of life. This is why engaging in advance care planning discussions is so important. It gives patients an opportunity to share their goals of care and values prior to incapacitation, and it gives you time to process this information, clarify and check your understanding, and feel confident in your decision-making on behalf of care partners down the line.

There are many forms and legal documents that are used to facilitate advance care planning. These include—though are not limited to—the healthcare proxy form, which identifies the person who will make decisions on behalf of the patient if there is a time when the patient is unable to make decisions for themselves, and Do-Not-Resuscitate (DNR) and Do-Not-Intubate (DNI) orders, which direct healthcare teams to withhold certain types of care. The phrase *advance medical directive* is an umbrella term for legal documents such as these which outline goals of care and how—ideally—they should be carried out. In Table 5.2, I've provided an overview of common documents used to help facilitate and record advanced care planning discussions. Importantly, like discussions about goals of care, advanced medical directives are not static; instead, these forms can be re-completed to reflect shifting goals and values. In fact, I encourage you each time you engage in a discussion about your loved one's goals of care to check in to see if any changes in their goals need to be reflected in changes to documents that have already been signed.

Table 5.2: Common Documents Used to Facilitate Advance Care Planning

Document	What is it?	How is it used?
Living Will	The living will specifies what type of medical treatment a patient wants in the future. Each state has a unique living will document, but all encompass the same ideas.	A living will can be created at any time, but it only becomes effective if your care partner is determined to have a terminal illness (that is, anticipated to die because of illness) or they are at the end of life and unable to speak for themself. The living will is then used by you (as the healthcare proxy) in making decisions about their care.

Document	What is it?	How is it used?
Healthcare Proxy Form	The healthcare proxy form designates the person who will make healthcare decisions on a patient's behalf in the case that they are unable to do so themself (for example, if they are in a coma).	A healthcare proxy form can be executed at any time, but like the living will, it only goes into effect if your care partner is unable to make decisions on their own behalf. The person designated as the healthcare proxy will be responsible for making medical decisions on the patient's behalf and carrying out the directives that are specified in the living will. In most cases, the healthcare proxy is the caregiver.
Do-Not-Resuscitate (DNR) Order	The DNR order instructs healthcare providers not to do cardiopulmonary resuscitation (CPR) if a patient's breathing stops or their heart stops beating. Patients are never required to sign a DNR order.	While your care partner can choose to sign/not sign a DNR order at any time, these are most frequently presented to families when patients are admitted to the hospital. Importantly, DNR status can be changed. It's very important for you to be aware of your care partner's DNR status since caregivers are often asked whether their loved ones have signed a DNR order or not.

Document	What is it?	How is it used?
Do-Not-Intubate (DNI) Order	The DNI order specifies whether, in addition to receiving CPR, a patient would want to have a breathing tube inserted (intubated) if their breathing stops or their heart stops beating. As with the DNR order, patients are not required to sign a DNI order.	While patients can choose to sign/not sign a DNI order at any time, these are most frequently presented to families when patients are admitted to the hospital. Importantly, patients can choose to change their DNI status. It's very important for you to be aware of your care partner's DNI status since caregivers are usually asked whether their loved ones have signed a DNI order or not.
Physician/ Medical Orders for Life-Sustaining Treatment (POLST/ MOLST)	POLST/MOLST forms address medical care for people with life-limiting illnesses. They include DNR/DNI status but are more comprehensive and cover additional treatments, such as antibiotic use and feeding tubes.	Your care partner should complete these forms if they are seriously ill or told that they have less than a year to live. If they are admitted to the hospital with a life-threatening condition, you (as the healthcare proxy) may be asked to complete these forms.
Power of Attorney	The power of attorney is a written authorization executed by the patient for someone to represent or act on their behalf in private affairs, business, or other legal matters.	While not central to the medical side of advance care planning discussions, caregivers are frequently designated as the power of attorney. This allows you to handle the administrative and financial side of care if your care partner is unable to do so due to illness or incapacitation.

The completion of advance medical directives is important for all patients and caregivers. However, these documents may be particularly important for sexual and gender minority (SGM) patients and caregivers who are chosen family members for one another. Chosen family members and partners with and without legal unions with SGM patients have not always been recognized as caregivers and healthcare proxies by both biological family members and healthcare providers.[9] At the same time, SGM patients historically have lower rates of completion of advance directives, including living wills and healthcare proxy forms.[10] Together, these factors can lead to situations in which patients' goals of care may be disregarded, their families of choice may be excluded from decision-making,[11] and undesignated families of origin are contacted to make healthcare decisions that may conflict with a patient's wishes.[12] These situations are not only detrimental to the care patients receive but can also have devastating effects on caregivers in bereavement. This lack of recognition of roles as healthcare proxies and chosen family members contributes to *disenfranchised grief*, that is, grief that is not acknowledged and validated.[13] For caregivers of SGM patients who are not formally recognized as chosen family and healthcare proxies, such grief can be profound and can contribute to isolation and mental health challenges.[14] For all these reasons, if you are a caregiver or chosen family member for an SGM patient, I encourage you to open a discussion about goals of care and advance directives with your loved one so that their goals of care can be carried forward down the line, and your role and efforts can be formally acknowledged.

It's Never Too Early
to Discuss Goals of Care

Many caregivers have shared with me their regretting how long they waited to engage in advance care planning discussions. Certainly, the idea of talking about goals of care soon after a loved one's initial diagnosis can feel premature. The conversation has the potential to be difficult for everyone and made even more challenging by feelings of anxiety and distress. However, avoiding these discussions endangers patients' ability to receive care that respects their wishes. Families often expect healthcare providers to initiate conversations, but healthcare providers frequently avoid frank and open dialogue about advance care planning or delay it until it is too late.[15] And even in cases when healthcare providers are discussing goals of care early on and repeatedly, what patients and caregivers each understand is not always consistent.

This was the case for Daniel, who came to me shortly before his husband Nathan's glioblastoma multiforme recurred. Gliobastoma is an aggressive brain tumor that received significant media attention after it took the life of John McCain. Like many caregivers of patients with brain tumors, there was a significant discrepancy in what Daniel and Nathan knew—or understood—about Nathan's prognosis. They both had been given the same information initially: Glioblastoma would never be cured, and the likelihood of long-term survival was low. But once Nathan completed chemotherapy and had a clean scan, he felt very strongly that he had "beat the cancer." Daniel, on the other hand, had become very knowledgeable about the statistics on recurrence and had participated in a monthly support group for caregivers of patients with glioblastoma in which he heard many stories of how quickly the tumor could return and, once back, how aggressive it could be.

Daniel desperately wanted to sit down with Nathan and have a conversation about what type of care he wanted in the future, at a time when (he knew it was *when*, not *if*) the tumor would return, and Nathan would potentially no longer be able to reliably communicate effectively. He was already his healthcare proxy but felt the weight of what could eventually be a tortuous decision to make. Each time Daniel attempted these conversations, Nathan vehemently resisted; he had become more irritable and verbally combative since his diagnosis, which his oncologist had normalized as part of potential tumor-related personality changes. In those moments, Daniel felt like he didn't know his husband; he had been calm and even-tempered for the thirty years of their relationship, rarely showing irritability or anger. Now, he was often downright mean to Daniel, even though Daniel was doing everything he could to take care of him. This was what Daniel called a "cruel punishment," being treated terribly by his husband at the time when he most needed his caring tone. It was this dynamic that eventually led him to seek support with me. During one of our first sessions, he told me something that has been echoed by many caregivers of patients with glioblastoma and other brain tumors: he felt like he had already lost his husband, since Nathan had changed so much from the tumor and he had already experienced multiple losses in their relationship.

Three months after Nathan completed chemotherapy, he suffered a massive seizure, and a subsequent scan showed that his glioblastoma had recurred. In the coming days, it became increasingly difficult for Nathan to engage in meaningful conversations. And, because of these changes, there was growing pressure on Daniel to take responsibility for healthcare communication. In the absence of their having clear conversations about goals of care earlier on, Daniel was not sure if it would be best to move forward with another aggressive treatment presented as one option by their oncologist or transition to more palliative-focused care. Nathan was sixty-eight, and they had had plans to enjoy their retirement years by traveling around the world. Their son was now an adult and living with his girlfriend, who Daniel believed would become his wife. Daniel knew Nathan wanted to be present for his son's wedding, and when he was first diagnosed, he feared that that might not be a possibility. In the absence of their having more conversations about goals of care before the recurrence of Nathan's cancer, and Nathan's initial expression early on after his diagnosis that they should try everything possible, they moved forward with the second-line treatment. This ultimately created more challenges to Nathan's quality of life, without a significant improvement in his life span. Following Nathan's death ten months after the cancer recurrence, Daniel shared regret for not having more open conversations with Nathan early on. He had been so concerned about upsetting him that he avoided important topics and eventually lost the window in which he was capable of meaningfully having these discussions.

In bereavement, our work focused in part on helping Daniel to see the role that Nathan had played in their communication, both before and after his glioblastoma diagnosis. Nathan had tended to be emotionally avoidant from the beginning of their relationship, and Daniel often felt responsible for opening important conversations throughout their life together, not just after Nathan was diagnosed. Gradually, Daniel acknowledged the longevity of this dynamic and the efforts he had made for many years to cultivate more open and productive communication. This framework allowed him to eventually adopt a kinder perspective on himself and what was and was not said to Nathan, and to look back on the effort he made to engage in difficult conversations with pride.

The Importance of Caregivers' Advocacy when Goals of Care Are Challenged

The open dialogue my dad and I had about advance care planning made the frequent questioning by multiple members of hospital healthcare teams after hearing his goals of care particularly distressing. I realize looking back now that many of these reactions likely reflected the perfect storm of ageism, as I discussed in the last chapter, with another major challenge to the current healthcare system and for countless caregivers: the challenge of disorders of consciousness. Disorders of consciousness are disorders that impact patients' abilities to be awake and aware. Knowledge about recovery of brain functioning among patients with disorders of consciousness has greatly advanced but has produced profound challenges for patients and caregivers who are often met with disbelief among healthcare professionals about patients' capacity for meaningful life. As Dr. Joseph Fins chronicles in *Rights Come to Mind: Brain Injury, Ethics, and the Struggle for Consciousness*,[16] while in some situations a loss of consciousness is either permanent or will limit recovery to a level that would be unacceptable to the person who is injured, many situations exist in which the appearance of these conditions belies a marked capacity to recover. That is, for many patients with disorders of consciousness, the ability to recover and experience meaningful functioning, connection, and communication exists but is met with significant doubt and challenge within our healthcare system. My dad's experience with fluctuations in consciousness due to Lewy body disease is a powerful example of this; such fluctuations leave patients periodically deeply unresponsive but nonetheless capable of emerging to enjoy years of meaningful life. At all times, my dad retained his zest for life, his short- and long-term memory, his creative ability to compose music and extraordinary prose, and yet, at any moment he could experience a fluctuation of consciousness and lose connection with our lived reality. This left me, as his caregiver, with the job of trying to convince his healthcare providers—many of whom had never witnessed Lewy body disease fluctuations before—of his capacity for recovery. Too often, it felt like no matter what I might say about what he was doing yesterday or the week or month before, what they saw in front of them *was* his permanent future and one that was utterly unchangeable. Moreover, knowing that he had Lewy body disease subsequently provided a backdrop for misinterpretation of symptoms that led to countless challenging, and even medically dangerous, moments.

One such occasion stands out to me. It was 2015, and one of the first times my dad was hospitalized after my mom died. He had a UTI (the most common driver of trips to the hospital were these infections), and while I always tried to be with him in the morning for the doctors' rounds, I had to give an important early morning presentation at work and couldn't make it on time. However, I checked in by phone shortly after with the medical resident who was assigned to his case. She shared with me that my dad couldn't interact meaningfully with the team when they rounded that morning, and as a result they wanted to have a goals-of-care conversation with me later that day in light of what was appearing to be worsening Lewy body disease.

While I am clearly *very* in favor of goals-of-care conversations, her suggestion of having one in that moment was so distressing to me. My dad's infection was under control, and I had just begun to discuss with the social worker his discharge home and getting him set up for physical and occupational therapy through the Visiting Nurse Service of New York. I had also just begun to schedule a handful of meetings for him with the librarians at the New York Public Library for the Performing Arts, where he was working on donating his music. There was life to be lived outside the hospital. Being asked to discuss goals of care in that emotional moment felt like code for *it's time to stop intervening, time to stop planning for the future.*

I ran from my apartment—which was approximately door-to-door 5.2 minutes away (a run I perfected over the years)—to my dad's bedside and found him lying on his side, his eyes closed, and his hands tightly gripping the bars of the hospital bed. He was practicing a deep breathing exercise he learned from one of his doctors to help him manage physical discomfort. I can imagine from the perspective of someone not familiar with my dad that he looked either like he was sleeping or in some sort of altered cognitive state. But I kissed his cheek and told him I loved him, and he opened his eyes. He was completely clearheaded and told me that he had pressed the call button repeatedly over the previous night because he needed his diaper to be changed, but no one came to change him. By the time the team rounded that morning, he was exhausted from no sleep and in great discomfort. That, combined with his inability to hear the questions being asked of him, led to a presentation that could very easily be perceived as disoriented.

Looking back, I can certainly empathize with the passing medical teams who questioned my dad's goals of care after they had witnessed him hallucinate for hours. Yet, when I was asked about his goals of care, what I shared was so frequently met with resistance. Over time, I noticed a pattern emerge with many of the rounding teams: They would ask me, repeatedly, whether my dad had signed a DNR order and whether we had discussed his goals of care. Eventually it felt as if my prior response, or what had been documented by the previous team in his medical record, was unsatisfying and that through repeated questioning they were pressuring me to change the answer. In fact, these repeated rounds of questioning did on occasion make me question my dad's goals and his—and my—intentions. Nonetheless, I shared, often verbatim, my dad's wishes for care and for his life.

If you are taking care of a patient who suffers from a disorder of consciousness, or from any illness that impacts their cognition and brain functioning and ability to advocate for themselves, you may face challenges in conveying their goals of care at some point. I want to normalize how difficult, frustrating, and intensely painful it can be to be questioned by members of the healthcare team. In these moments, it's easy to question yourself; I certainly did. However, as long as you have had clear discussions with your care partner about their goals, what you are conveying to members of the healthcare team are exactly that: *their goals*. One step I took that was helpful in reinforcing my confidence in conveying my dad's goals of care is (with his permission) I periodically audio recorded our conversations. Then, in moments when he was fluctuating and I was being questioned about his goals, I would be able to listen back to these recordings to reinforce what I was advocating for. Whether it's audio or video recordings, jotting down notes, or telling a trusted friend about the conversation soon after it happens, anything you can do to document these conversations will help to boost your confidence in your advocacy, especially if you are met with questions and challenges by members of the healthcare team.

❋   ❋   ❋

In June of 2018, my dad sustained his first and only fall at home. He slipped while in the shower with the home health aide. He suffered only minor injuries, but we took him, regardless, for evaluation in the ER. The next morning, a senior attending geriatrician who had taken care of my dad in 2013 when he was in the coma happened to be rounding. My dad was approximately fifty pounds heavier than he was when he first presented to this doctor in 2013, and he was fully awake, engaged, strong, oriented, and his immensely charming self. After they spoke, she shared with me how amazing it was to have the opportunity to get to know my dad, and how grateful she was that I had held on to hope and continued to advocate for him and his goals over the past five years. No doubt, this advocacy helped to give him those five extra years of life.

There is no one-size-fits-all goals-of-care plan. There is no one right answer to the question, "What would be a good or meaningful death?" just as there is no one right answer to the question, "What does meaningful life mean to you?" As we humans are unique, so, too, are our goals of care, our goals for life, and death. I did not share our story to imply that DNR orders are harmful; on the contrary, they often have profound benefits to patients and caregivers. Additionally, I don't mean to suggest that advance care planning can only be effectively carried out when there exists the type of relationship I had with my dad. These conversations can be navigated productively even in the context of strained family relationships. However, I am certain that had I not had open, vulnerable, and repeated conversations with my dad about what was important to him at critical junctures during his illness trajectory, I would not have been able to make decisions that were in line with his goals and values. I would not have been able to help him have a few extra years of life during which he was able to enjoy many important milestones, and I would not have been able to help him have an end-of-life experience that was as close as realistically possible to his goals.

So many of the challenges that we face—as patients, caregivers, and healthcare providers—in engaging in advance care planning stem from our discomfort with talking about death. Undoubtedly, in the United States, talking about death and dying is taboo. It's not something that is an accepted part of our national dialogue, or at least it hasn't been for most of my life. And inevitably, this avoidance intensifies the unhelpful thoughts and feelings we all have about talking about death.

Like my patient Daniel, who came to accept his husband's role in their difficulty discussing goals of care, it's also necessary to acknowledge the significant role played by healthcare professionals in these discussions. Navigating these conversations cannot be the sole responsibility of patients and caregivers. Graduate medical education must do a better job of teaching all new healthcare professionals to sensitively discuss death and dying, to effectively discuss advance care planning, and more broadly, to appreciate the wide variety of goals of care patients have. Even when you have put the tools I've suggested to use, have become seasoned at healthcare communication, and have a clear understanding of your care partner's goals of care, engaging with healthcare professionals who inadequately or insensitively address this topic undermines the work you will have done. Improving the training of all healthcare providers in sensitive communication skills, including cultivating their capacity to follow the Platinum Rule[17] and simultaneously hold their goals and values and those of the patient without letting one overshadow the other, will improve their capacity to provide personalized care and assist with preserving the dignity of patients and caregivers.

That is my hope for the future. For now, I hope that you are thinking about your own answer to the question, "What would be a good or meaningful death?" Taking time to think through this question is a powerful exercise. It's never too early to answer this question, and it's never too early to ask it of those we love.

CHAPTER 6

The Caregiving House of Cards

A Little Bit of Everything

Artist: Joanie Sommers
Produced and Arranged by Stan Applebaum, 1963

It was three in the afternoon, and I was sitting with my sixth patient of the day. During the five minutes I had between patients, I checked my phone and saw several missed calls: one from the Visiting Nurse Service of New York's main number, one from an unknown number but what I suspected to be that of the nurse assigned to come visit my dad that afternoon, one from my dad's pharmacy, and one from the Center for Disability Rights, the organization that assisted with my dad's access to Medicaid coverage. I also had multiple texts from my dad's home health aide detailing the current issue with a leaky catheter, pictures of the empty urine collection bag, and my dad's latest vital signs—that is, his blood pressure, oxygen saturation, and temperature. These were all normal so I felt safe waiting the two more hours before I would finish sessions and be able to take more than a minute to respond. I took a deep inhale and tried to orient myself to the present moment, tucking away the racing thoughts I had about what I needed to do as soon as the session ended to focus completely on the patient sitting across from me.

From 2013 until my dad's death in 2019, this was my daily caregiving house of cards, the balancing act all caregivers are asked to perform that takes immense energy and resources and is inherently fragile and precarious without external support. At all times I was balancing my professional identity and commitment to work with that of my responsibilities as my dad's caregiver, the latter of which involved what seemed like multiple identities.

Caregivers have always been the backbone of our healthcare system, concurrently playing the role of partner, parent, child, sibling, or friend, and physician, nurse, social worker, lawyer, and patient navigator. While I had just finished my PhD a few years before I transitioned into the caregiving role, it eventually felt as if I earned my degree as a seasoned social worker and even nurse and lawyer and financial planner in the context of my caregiving journey. The skills I needed to carry out the medical and nursing responsibilities of caregiving, to carry out the physical, financial, legal, ethical, and social responsibilities of caregiving, molded me into a caregiving superhero who had access to the expertise of all these professions. We all as humans at times must juggle multiple responsibilities. But the act of building and supporting this house of cards to take care of the medically ill or disabled, perhaps more than any other, is one that asks of us to develop a multitude of skills in the absence of formal training. So much of the burden and distress caregivers report is the downstream effect of these responsibilities, for which most of us receive minimal to no support. Looking back, it's striking that in the context of all these responsibilities handed to us, there are no correlates of baby showers or childbirth classes for new caregivers wherein support and supplies are provided. We do dramatically more to help families bringing humans into this world than to help caregivers supporting family members who are making their exit.

My personal and professional experiences have highlighted several categories of responsibilities that are particularly challenging, and which often come as a surprise: These include handling significant medical and nursing tasks, facilitating case management, and serving as a family mediator. By drawing attention to these responsibilities, I hope to make them less surprising to you so that, when you're challenged, you will feel more prepared.

Caregivers as Healthcare Professionals

Nearly all of you will, at some point, perform medical or nursing tasks as part of your caregiving responsibilities. My guess is for those of you who've already been caregivers, you have done these things without sufficient education or support. For me, the medical and nursing side of caregiving was prominent and included: taking my dad's vital signs (temperature, blood oxygen level, pulse, and blood pressure); administering oral (in the form of pills) and subcutaneous (that is, injectable) medications; changing the bags for—and cleaning the opening to—his suprapubic catheter; monitoring the amount and color of the urine output in his catheter bags, always keeping my eyes out for visible signs of infections, such as his urine being cloudy or bloody; and administering eye drops each night (after weeks in a coma my dad suffered significant drying of his eyes, which never seemed to fully resolve). There were other responsibilities I had during times when he was being treated for pressure ulcers or other skin infections like cellulitis or other specific ailments. While our home health aides were all trained in these tasks, it was only in the last months of my dad's life that he had twenty-four-hour care, so for years, the above were at many times my responsibilities. Thinking back, I never once received any formal training to do any of these tasks. Thanks to digital machines, taking my dad's vital signs wasn't difficult, though the blood pressure cuff and pulse oximeter were often unreliable. As a result, I eventually learned to take blood pressure readings the old-fashioned way with a stethoscope after repeatedly requesting impromptu training from one of the visiting nurses. I learned to administer injectable medications to help with his anemia, and admittedly the first time I prepared to give the injection it took at least ten minutes for me to get the courage to do so (he was such a good sport). I learned on the job, as all caregivers do, and the learning curve was steep. By the end of my caregiving journey, I had become a highly attuned diagnostician, could identify the early signs of UTI or dehydration, could stage a bedsore and implement the proper wound care routine, and knew all the drug and food interactions for my dad's medication regimen. I had a keen understanding of the risks of IV fluids on my dad's cardiac functioning and knew to watch for swelling of his legs as a sign of heart failure. I could interpret basic blood panels and advise on which antibiotics worked best for the type of bacteria that showed up in his urine culture. I had taken an informal course in internal medicine while on the job and seemed to have passed the final exam.

I'm not alone in this.

Almost every caregiver I've worked with has had to, at some point, take responsibility for medical or nursing tasks, and very often, without much training to do so. These range from simple tasks like giving oral medications to the more complex tasks, like the responsibilities of my patient Florence, whose husband, Michael, had been diagnosed with an acute myeloid leukemia (AML) and had been cleared to undergo an outpatient autologous hematopoietic cell transplantation. Traditionally, patients are admitted to the hospital for an extensive inpatient stay before and after transplants, due to treatment toxicities and high risk for infectious complications. More recently, in part because of the challenges experienced by patients who remain isolated in inpatient settings for months at a time, combined with the financial cost and burden on the healthcare system and the desire to reduce hospital-induced infections, new protocols have been implemented that allow certain patients to return to their home immediately after the transplant. These protocols have many benefits to patients, families, and our healthcare system, but such benefits come at a significant cost to caregivers like Florence: enrollment in these transplants often requires the consent of caregivers to be available for twenty-four hours a day, seven days a week, for at least two weeks to a month after the initial transplant, and for extended periods of time through the first hundred days post-transplant.

This is an enormous responsibility. Caregivers are required to maintain sterility of the home or homelike setting (many families opt to stay in temporary apartments near the hospital), knowing that the introduction of pathogens from something as simple as an undercooked vegetable could be life threatening. They are also required to monitor patients for signs and symptoms of a variety of adverse events and generally serve as the eyes and ears of the medical team. Translation: *Caregivers are asked to serve as the ad hoc nursing staff.*

Florence had come to me for support when Michael was initially diagnosed with AML, but it was his enrollment in the homebound transplant program that led to a significant increase in her distress. She felt incredible pressure from her family and the medical team to be "on call," checking on her husband at all times of day and night for signs of the transplant going awry. She constantly checked his temperature, his fluid intake and output, and symptoms like fatigue and nausea. She shared feeling scared that her attempts to maintain cleanliness in the home were imperfect. She cleaned every surface in their apartment, every place he sat, everything he touched. Florence was also responsible for cooking and helping her husband to maintain a special diet. She felt completely unprepared for how much her husband was going to deteriorate after the transplant, and for the magnitude of care he would require. Perhaps more than any caregiver with whom I've worked, Florence had been given extensive training by her husband's medical team to prepare her for the responsibilities she would have at home, but nonetheless, she felt completely overwhelmed with what was on her shoulders. She went into the transplant period committed to maintaining a work-from-home schedule, but eventually took time off via FMLA and then went to part-time work because she felt physically incapable of doing everything her husband required, in addition to her own work.

Florence's experience is not a unique one. Over the past decade, there has been a dramatic shift in the United States to out-of-hospital care. This shift has been met with significant financial savings and in many cases, superior outcomes for patients who are at risk for hospital-acquired infections and other adverse events while hospitalized. Yet this shift places significant demands on caregivers to shoulder what once were the responsibilities of trained healthcare professionals. These demands were movingly described in Kate Washington's memoir, *Already Toast: Caregiving and Burnout in America*.[1] Like Florence, Kate was assumed to have the skills, ability, and willingness to take care of all her husband's needs upon his discharge home, including, for example, administering IV antibiotics three times a day through a PICC (peripherally inserted central catheter) line that went from his arm to his heart. She ultimately was unprepared both for the magnitude of tasks required as well as the potential complications and medical trajectory that her husband eventually experienced.

Across diagnoses, caregivers describe their loved one's discharge from the hospital to home as the most anxiety-provoking experience because of all the new responsibilities they are asked to assume, those that are traditionally performed by medical staff *in* the hospital. And, in the past decade, there has been a pronounced increase in these responsibilities, without a correlate increase in training. This represents an issue that requires immediate attention. As caregivers in the nursing role, your loved ones' lives are very often in your hands. It is an incredible responsibility. As it is for so many caregivers, my dad's discharge to home was always an intensely stressful time for me, as it meant a new responsibility, a new skill I would need to pick up, an additional step added to a daily nursing routine.

In addition to these predominantly medical tasks, like Florence and Kate and so many of the caregivers who have sought care in the clinic, I ultimately assisted with nursing tasks that challenged both me and my dad on a deep existential level. For us, that task was my changing his diapers. I remember the first time this happened. It was in the early summer of 2014 and my dad was staying at my apartment overnight as he often did after having his catheter changed at the hospital nearby. The home health aide had gotten him showered, changed, and safely in bed before he left at 8:30 that evening, but about a half hour later my dad felt his stomach rumble and asked if we could get the aide to come back. He knew that he was going to have a bowel movement, and he knew that remaining in a soiled diaper overnight would be uncomfortable, unsafe, and, in his words, not fair to me, as he was sleeping in my bed. I texted our aide, but he was already on a train home to Queens.

I sat at the side of the bed holding my dad's hand, while he teared up and shared that my changing his diaper was the last thing he would ever want me to do, the last thing he would ever think of putting me through. It was an intensely painful and difficult moment for us both, as it was also the *last* thing I, as his daughter, ever wanted to do. Not only was I unsure of how I would physically be able to do it (I had watched the aides multiple times maneuver my dad using disposable bed pads called "chucks" but hadn't ever done this myself) but I had also tried in the context of our experiences as partners in care to preserve my dad's dignity and this one very intimate boundary, that I now was about to cross. We talked a bit more about the absurdity of the situation, his tears turned slowly to laughter, and I turned on classical music so that we could have a distraction. I got out the chucks and a basin with water and soap, put on latex gloves, quickly drank a small glass of wine (perhaps the only time in my life I've ever truly needed liquid courage was that night), and proceeded to roll my dad onto his side to undo his diaper, holding his full weight with my right arm while I shoved a chuck underneath his hips with my left. I repeated the procedure on his other side and eventually freed him of the soiled diaper and was left with the task of cleaning him, making sure to avoid the partially healed bedsore on his sacrum. I then once again rolled him on his left side to begin the process of putting on a fresh diaper, which I found much more complicated than the initial diaper removal, and realized why, when I had witnessed staff in the hospital do this, they always worked in pairs. This was thoroughly complicated and physically challenging.

Throughout the process I did my best to maintain as much eye contact as possible with my dad to help him to feel a little less vulnerable. I did not want him to sense what I was inevitably feeling inside, aside from incompetence: sadness and disgust. Sadness that he was so physically limited and helpless, and yes, disgust, that I was cleaning feces out of his genital area. An awful feeling to experience but a very real one, and one shared by so many of the caregivers with whom I've worked.

We are tasked as caregivers at times to do things—like changing the diapers or colostomy bags of our adult parents or romantic partners—that go against the very essence of what defines the nature of our relationship. And yet we do these things because we have no choice. We do them because we love, and we care. The emotional price tag of performing these tasks, however, can be substantial. My dad was ashamed, and I felt disgust. While certainly the experience connected us on a deeper level and engendered a new degree of bidirectional respect, it stands out as one of the more difficult moments in our journey. His life wasn't at stake that night, but the innocence of our relationship as father and daughter was.

The feelings that I had that night were very normal. If you find yourself in a similar situation, it will be helpful for you to acknowledge the feelings that come up for you, whatever they are, and even share them with a trusted friend or therapist. As caregivers, we are adept at being hard on ourselves, and again and again I hear stories of caregivers who judged themselves for having feelings such as disgust or resentment, with thoughts like, "I'm a terrible person for feeling this way about her." If you find yourself doing this, I want you to imagine what a close friend might say to you. See if, instead of judging yourself, you might be able to choose to focus on feeling proud of yourself for doing some of the most difficult work of caregiving.

Caregivers as Case Managers

A second category of responsibility that is immensely overwhelming, and may take you by surprise, is case management. Case managers are paid employees within health systems who work to facilitate patient care by assessing patient needs, evaluating treatment options, creating treatment plans, coordinating care, and gauging progress. As a caregiver, you will most likely be asked to assume many case management responsibilities at home without pay, including: coordinating medical appointments and facilitating communication between different healthcare professionals and institutions; determining what changes need to be made at home to make the home safe for your care partner, such as installing shower chairs, grab bars, and ramps; and navigating the financial side of healthcare, such as figuring out how to pay for care delivered by physicians, as well as by other professionals like home health aides.

To help you be as prepared as possible for the financial aspects of your future case management responsibilities, in Exercise 6.1 I provide a list of questions for you to ask your care partner and other members of your caregiving network. These questions would have been helpful for me to think through earlier on and to discuss with my parents when they were both alive, long in advance of my dad's complete dependence on others for care. Exploring these questions now will help to make the process of facilitating care in the future a bit easier for all involved, especially if your loved one will receive home health or nursing home care.

Exercise 6.1: Questions to Facilitate Caregivers' Roles as Case Managers

Questions for Caregivers to Ask Care Partners

- What health insurance do you have (e.g., Medicare, Medicaid, Blue Cross Blue Shield)? Do you have a secondary health insurance? If so, what benefits does it provide?
- What home care services, if any, are covered by your current health insurance plan(s)?
- Do you have a long-term care policy? If so, how much money currently remains in that policy?
- Do you have savings put away that can be used to pay for medical care and home healthcare services? If so, how much is available?

- What is your total annual income? Income includes everything from payments from employers, to pensions and Social Security payments, as well as investments.
- Do you qualify today for Medicaid? If not, how much above your state's Medicaid limit is your current income?
- Do I have access to all your bank accounts? If not, what steps can we take now to ensure that I have access?
- Am I your power of attorney? If not, what steps can be taken so that I can be designated as your power of attorney?

Questions for Caregivers to Ask Themselves

- What funds do I have available to help pay for my loved one's care?
- To what extent will using my own funds impact my ability to live comfortably, both now and in the future?
- Are there any additional sources of funds from other family and friends that can be used to help offset the cost of care?

These questions are important ones because, like the emotional and physical effects of caregiving, the financial effects are equally dramatic and enduring. As with many caregivers, the long-term financial impact of caregiving was not at the forefront of my mind when my dad was here. I never questioned my choice of using my salary to take care of him, but I realize in retrospect how this selfless act has been detrimental for my future. Only now have I been finally able to begin to build, and I am acutely aware that I lost out on nearly a decade of savings. The financial reverberations of my caregiving journey are loud and will last my lifetime, as they do for so many others.

Importantly, your role as a case manager will be facilitated by your being designated formally as both your care partner's healthcare proxy and power of attorney. It can also be helpful to have your care partner share their consent to have you involved in healthcare conversations, appointment scheduling, and related matters with members of their healthcare team.

Caregivers as Mediators

One of the most important elements of your caregiving journey is your relationship with your partner in care and with others in the family and caregiving network. These relationships have the potential to deeply shape your experience of caregiving, from how you feel emotionally to the logistic and financial challenges you face. Caregivers frequently become the point person for sharing healthcare information with a wide network of family and friends, a responsibility which can be intensely stressful. As the hub of this information-flow wheel, you will likely need to navigate balancing the varied emotional needs of many.

This was the case for Nicolas, who came to see me a few months after his mother, Sofia, was diagnosed with esophageal cancer. Nicolas was twenty-six and single, and lived alone ten minutes away from his mother in the Bronx. Nicolas's father had died when Nicolas was a child, and he had been raised primarily by his mother and older sister, Elena, who was thirty-seven and lived in New Jersey with her husband and two children. Their extended family—Nicolas's aunts, uncles, and cousins—all lived in the Dominican Republic. When their mother was first diagnosed and underwent surgery, both Nicolas and Elena accompanied her to her medical appointments and assisted with her recovery at home. English was Sofia's second language, and she depended on her children to clarify and often translate information shared with her by the medical team into Spanish. After Sofia recovered and began a long series of radiation treatments, Elena made it clear that it would be too difficult for her to commute more than once a week to the Bronx and that Nicolas would need to step in to manage most of the care. This was infuriating to Nicolas, who had been working two jobs to make ends meet and help take care of his mom long before her cancer diagnosis. Nicolas felt that as the man of the house, it was important that he support his mom, but deep down he harbored resentment for Elena for not contributing more. Nicolas felt abandoned. Added to these feelings was his new responsibility of keeping Sofia's extended family in the Dominican Republic up to date on her medical condition and treatments. Throughout the week he fielded phone calls and texts from his uncle, aunt, and cousins, all of whom repeatedly called his phone if their texts weren't immediately answered. Over time, it seemed like Nicolas's extended family began looking to him for emotional support; each request for information was followed by an implicit request for reassurance that Sofia would survive. Instead of receiving gratitude from his extended family for all he was doing, Nicolas often felt blamed for his mom's disease progression. And the icing on the cake for him was that not once did any of his extended family members ask him how he was doing, or what they could do to help.

Our work together during this time focused, in part, on helping Nicolas to understand how beneath the anger he felt from his extended family was likely sadness, fear, and powerlessness. It is generally easier to express anger than sadness, and beneath anger one can usually discover a deep well of sadness. This framework did not immediately mitigate the resentment Nicolas felt about his family not coming to help in New York ("If they felt so badly, why didn't they just come here?" he ruminated), but it did help soften the feelings of hurt that were elicited in the presence of their anger. Imagining their sadness and fear engendered within him a new sense of empathy for what they might be feeling. I also encouraged Nicolas to examine the thoughts he had during these interactions ("They are angry at me for Mom getting sicker"), and to remember that his family ultimately was not angry at him but instead at the disease. Externalizing cancer from his mom and himself was a powerful cognitive reframe that not only liberated him emotionally in subsequent interactions with his extended family but helped him to speak more openly to Sofia about his sadness. "I'm so angry at cancer for doing this to you, Mom," he shared with her shortly after this session.

We discussed ways in which Nicolas spent emotional energy, time spent resenting his sister and extended family and feeling intensely frustrated. This was emotional energy Nicolas did not have the luxury to expend. We explored ways in which he could reinvest the energy in himself and how he could use the feeling of resentment—which became a daily experience—as a reminder to check in with himself about what, if anything, he could do to make his day better.

Our work subsequently focused on what Nicolas did have control over: how he spent his time with his mom. Nicolas realized that despite the challenges it presented, caregiving gave him the opportunity to spend precious time with Sofia he would otherwise have not had.

Caregiving in the Context of Difficult Relationships

The emotional dynamics that are amplified when a family member gets sick are generally those that have been long-standing. Resentment between siblings, unrealistic or unfair expectations of elders, and preexisting marital difficulties are magnified when illness and caregiving are thrown into the mix. In fact, illness and caregiving in many ways form the ultimate test on relationships and family structures. Sibling relationships that were at baseline cordial like the one between Nicolas and Elena can either soften or become cold, transactional, and even hostile. Marital relationships that were once filled with love, physical intimacy, and warmth can endure or cool off to the point of freezing. Illness and caregiving are like a bright spotlight shined underneath a bed, where once-hidden early life emotional injuries, resentments, and fears come out of the woodwork.

The roles we play as caregivers in these emotional dynamics often reflect the roles we have always played in our family system, including that of family mediator. By family mediator, I mean the family member who finds themself working to soothe others, mending hurt feelings, and attempting to align family members' perspectives. The person who works to "keep the peace." This is invisible labor added on top of many other responsibilities that can powerfully shape your entire experience of caregiving. It's difficult enough to balance taking care of the medical, nursing, logistic, and financial elements of care without being asked to give often nonexistent emotional energy to others. But rarely do these responsibilities occur in an emotional vacuum. Like Nicolas, you may become the target of emotions that have absolutely nothing to do with you: anger, sadness, and legacies of hurt can get projected onto you and make an already-challenging caregiving role even more intense.

Many of you may also be tasked with taking care of someone with whom you have a difficult or even hostile relationship. For example, several patients of mine have been adult children taking care of parents who had previously been emotionally, physically, or verbally abusive to them, or who had abandoned them earlier in their life. Others were partners and spouses on the verge of separation but who felt boxed into caregiving—and the partnership—because of illness. Inevitably, a significant additional challenge for all these caregivers was navigating resentment, the emotional complexity of the preexisting dynamics, and ways in which it manifested in the caregiver–care partner relationship. Certainly, the term "loved one" will not accurately characterize all your care partners. I'm acutely aware that my caregiving experience was dramatically shaped by the fact that my care partner was also my best friend and how it would have likely been more challenging if it was anyone else in my life.

While we cannot choose the emotional tone of our family and our caregiver–care partner relationship at the time we step into this role, we can choose how to respond to existing challenges and limitations. Regardless of what type of relationship you have or will have with your care partner, members of your family, and broader care network, there are things that you can do to buffer negative emotions, protect yourself, and yes, capitalize on caregiving as an opportunity to improve these relationships.

First, while we can't change the past and the events leading up to the existing emotional dynamics between you, your care partner, and other family members, clear communication about how you are feeling can assist you to address current dynamics that are making your challenging caregiving role even more so. The XYZ technique is a simple way for you to think about framing your communication, whether it is about airing grievances or expressing appreciation. It encourages you to use only "I statements," not "You statements," and to avoid blame in communicating over a difficult issue.[2] The XYZ technique goes like this:

X: "I feel (or felt) ___X___"
Y: "When you say/do (or said/did) ___Y___"
Z: "Because ___Z___"

When I taught Nicolas the XYZ technique, he was able to use it with his sister, Elena, to address how hurt he felt, saying, "I felt really abandoned when you told me that it's too hard for you to come to the Bronx more than once a week, because for decades I've been taking responsibility for Mom, and we really should be a team here." The XYZ technique allows you to clearly state what you're feeling and why. It allows your family member to understand what specifically it is they are or aren't doing that's leading you to feel hurt. Certainly, it takes courage and vulnerability to share how you're feeling using this technique, and inevitably, the only person you have control over is you, meaning once you share how you feel, you cannot control how the other person will react. But keeping emotional wounds hidden is going to make everything feel worse.

You may find that the XYZ technique is not immediately effective. That is, the first time you use it, you might not get the desired response from the person you're speaking to. Many caregivers have found that they need to repeat themselves a few times before their messages are digested, before other members of the care network understand how their actions and words have been hurtful. Remember, when you open the dialogue, you will have already been preparing to have the discussion, while the person you're speaking to may be caught off guard. In my experience, simply repeating the XYZ technique may be enough to get your point across and eventually lead to some behavioral change.

Second, like with Nicolas, I encourage you to draw on the cognitive restructuring technique that I introduced in Chapter 3 to help maximize the ways you respond to difficult emotional dynamics in your family. As a reminder, there are three steps to this process:

First, identify the thoughts you're having that are associated with difficult emotions. For example, after his uncle expressed anger at him for his shortcomings as a caregiver and a man, Nicolas had thoughts like, "I'm failing my family—my mom's family—because she's getting sicker." His uncle's anger brought out feelings of shame.

Second, evaluate the evidence supporting the thoughts associated with difficult emotions. I encouraged Nicolas to explore the evidence that his thought was true or untrue and whether there was any alternative explanation. Nicolas was able to recognize that the harsh words from his uncle that led to these thoughts were driven by his uncle's own feelings of sadness and powerlessness. Instead of powerless, on days he didn't speak to his uncle, Nicolas felt like he was doing everything he could to take care of his mom and knew that he ultimately had no control over whether Sofia's cancer would spread.

The **third** step in cognitive restructuring is to **develop an alternative and more helpful thought**, such as "My uncle is sad because his sister is dying, but I am not responsible here. I'm doing the best that I can. In fact, I'm stepping up to be the man of the house in the way I know my dad would have wanted." This alternative thought brought out a deep sense of pride in Nicolas. It also inspired him to use the XYZ technique to tell his uncle how he was feeling: "Uncle, I feel really hurt when you tell me that I'm not doing enough, because I've given everything I have to give to Mom."

Cognitive restructuring is a powerful approach to coping with difficult emotions that come up in the context of complicated family dynamics, but sometimes the only "thing" for us to do to handle difficult family interactions—and yes, difficult family members—is breathe. Our breath is perhaps our most consistently powerful stress-management tool. Using the exercise I provided at the end of Chapter 3 as a guide, taking a deep diaphragmatic breath before responding to family members can give you a moment to pause and think about what it is you really want to say, and what is going to be most effective to say. This deep breath—in through your nose, held for a few seconds, and out through your mouth—brings oxygen to your brain and lowers your stress hormone cortisol, making it easier for you to respond in a calm and rational manner. Taking this breath also gives you a chance to evaluate the thoughts you are having and restructure any in the moment that might be unhelpful. Ultimately, these deep breaths will allow you to do what is most important: conserve your emotional energy.

Finally, for couples, families, and caregiving units who are struggling to navigate difficult emotions, and when such emotions negatively impact your ability to provide care and even the medical well-being of the patient, seeking the support of a trained mental health professional can be invaluable. Often just a handful of couples or family therapy sessions can powerfully address the dynamics arising. While as caregivers we often do take on the role of family mediator, giving that responsibility to a professional can help you to take a step back and focus more on the underlying relationships you have with your care partner and care network that are shaping your experience of caregiving.

*   *   *

Many caregivers have a wish, though it is one that is very rarely spoken aloud and often only within the safety of close friendships or therapy appointments: the wish for these responsibilities to end. A wish to no longer be relied on, to no longer be the point person among healthcare professionals and family members. A wish to be able to turn the ringer on their phone off. A wish to go to sleep without being on high alert for something bad happening with their care partner overnight. A wish to be able to save a paycheck or spend it on a vacation or a massage instead of on adult diapers and home health aides. A wish to make a plan for the future that they know they can keep. A wish to escape caregiving obligations and be free.

Like disgust and resentment, for many caregivers, these types of thoughts are often followed by judgment. I, too, had thoughts like these and then would emotionally punish myself for having them, given that the end of my caregiving responsibilities would ultimately mean the end of my dad's life. And yet, it would be impossible for any of us to shoulder such tremendous responsibilities and *not* have this type of thought, at least once.

Moments when these thoughts arise are phenomenal opportunities to think about ways in which you can better meet your needs, despite your current limitations. Given your responsibilities, you're very likely giving up a lot of your own life goals and dreams, or at least pressing pause on them. You might not be able to take that big trip you were hoping to take. You might not be able to take that job across the country that was attractive to you. You might not be able to save financially for your future. But despite these very real challenges, each of you can likely think of ways in which you can better meet your needs. This can be as simple as carving out a small amount of time every few days for exercise or planning for a weekend—or even just a day—away from your care partner so that you can get a breather. While certainly other very important life goals may remain on hold, doing everything you can to preserve yourself, each day, is the best way you can be a caregiver to yourself.

CHAPTER 7

Team Sports

Where the Boys Are

Artist: Connie Francis
Conducted and Arranged by Stan Applebaum, 1961

Caregivers are the long-term care system in the United States.

Yes, you read that correctly. As of today (2023), we do not have a social insurance program such as those available in countries like Germany and Japan that provide long-term care services. Which means that support for you and your caregiving responsibilities is extremely limited in this country. Unless you have a large network of family and friends who can assist you with taking care of a loved one, you are likely to rely at some point on the assistance of direct care workers, such as personal care aides, home health aides, and certified nursing assistants. Undoubtedly, the home healthcare workforce has become a somewhat invisible but critical element of the caring infrastructure in the United States.

In this chapter, I describe who direct care workers are, what they do, and how you can go about securing their assistance. Caregivers will frequently share with me that they wish they had employed a direct care worker much earlier because of the significant and positive impact such individuals ultimately had on so many aspects of their and their care partners' lives. At the same time, figuring out how to find and employ direct care workers who you can afford, who have the skills necessary to meet your loved one's healthcare needs, and with whom you and your care partner feel comfortable can feel like finding a needle in a haystack. My hope is that this chapter will bring awareness to the invaluable work done by direct care workers and provide you with guidance to assist you in involving them on your care team.

✳   ✳   ✳

In 2016, I noticed a small, red, slightly itchy and painful circle in the inner crease of my elbow. Within twenty-four hours, a thin red streak began to crawl from that mark up toward my armpit. A quick Google search revealed that this was likely one of three things, the most concerning of which was cellulitis, a potentially serious bacterial skin infection. I was familiar with cellulitis, as my dad had suffered several such infections on his legs in the past, and I knew that the heat radiating from my arm was similar to that from his legs when he had been sick. I went to the urgent care center that was conveniently located next to my dad's building, and within minutes I was told to go immediately to the emergency room, that my own health was at significant risk.

In typical caregiver fashion, I ignored the first part of that advice and went directly to my dad's bedside, where I shared with him the news of my potential cellulitis infection and the directions I was given to go to the hospital. I quickly put out seven days' worth of his standing medications and sent a group text to all the home health aides involved in his care, letting them know that I would likely be unavailable for several days. The weight of my upcoming absence felt heavy on my shoulders, and I scrambled to find backup care should an emergency occur during my absence, either with my dad or one of the aides. And then I got myself quickly to the hospital, where I was immediately admitted.

The nurse who evaluated me when I arrived in the ER gave me an inquisitive look as he took my history; he recognized that a little over a week earlier I had stood by my dad in a stretcher in that same room. We realized that my cellulitis infection had likely begun when I picked up bacteria during that hospital admission, and the fact that the intervening week was one of many sleepless nights and high stress made my body more susceptible and weakened my immune system's capacity to fight off the infection. This was caregiver burden at its finest.

If I had been living in a different era, perhaps that of my grandparents or great-grandparents in Eastern Europe before World War I, it is likely that my absence at home during my hospital admission would have been easily compensated for by a multigenerational family system that would have stepped in to provide care. Today in the United States, such multigenerational homes, in which three or even four generations of family members reside, are the exception rather than the norm. Instead, we increasingly rely on the invaluable assistance of home health aides and other direct care workers to provide care to patients at home, and by extension, their families.

This was the case for my family. After several very challenging stays in a rotation of nursing homes in 2013, when my dad and I revisited his goals of care after my mom died, he was adamant about avoiding nursing homes altogether. In order to respect his wishes and make it possible for him to remain at home, without an extended family network that could step in to help, and in the absence of my own physical capacity to provide all the care that my dad required, we relied heavily on the assistance of home health aides. Without them, it would have been impossible for me to honor my dad's wishes.

Who Are Direct Care Workers?

Broadly, direct care workers assist individuals with activities of daily living (ADLs) and instrumental activities of daily living (IADLs), the tasks that I described in Chapter 2. There are currently 4.7 million direct care workers who serve as the paid front line of support for patients and their families, and a total of 7.9 million total direct care job openings are anticipated by 2030.[1] This represents more new jobs than any other occupation in the United States.

In Table 7.1, I provide an overview of the various classifications in the direct care workforce and the types of tasks they perform.

Table 7.1: Classification of Direct Care Workers[2]

Title	Description and scope of work
Direct Care Worker	Assists older adults and people with disabilities with daily tasks and activities across LTSS,* hospitals, and other settings. Direct care workers are formally classified as personal care aides, home health aides, and nursing assistants, but their specific job titles vary according to where they work and the populations they serve.
Home Care Worker	An aggregate term for direct care workers—primarily personal care aides and home health aides—who provide assistance to individuals in their own homes.

---

* LTSS (Long-Term Services and Supports): a range of health and social services provided to individuals who require assistance with ADLs and IADLs. Also described as long-term care.

Title	Description and scope of work
Home Health Aide	Direct care worker who provides ADL and IADL assistance to individuals in the community and who may also perform certain clinical tasks under the supervision of a licensed professional.
Independent Provider	Direct care worker who is employed directly by consumers through publicly funded consumer-directed programs or private-pay arrangements.
Nursing Assistant	Direct care worker who provides ADL and IADL assistance, as well as completes certain clinical tasks, for individuals living in skilled nursing homes.
Personal Care Aide	Direct care worker who assists individuals with ADLs and/or IADLs in their homes and communities, and who may also support individuals with employment and other forms of community engagement.
Residential Care Aide	Direct care worker who assists individuals living in adult family homes, assisted living communities, and other community-based residential care settings.
Direct Support Professional	Direct care worker who assists individuals with intellectual and developmental disabilities across a range of settings.

As a caregiver, you are likely to encounter various types of direct care workers described in Table 7.1, especially if your loved one is admitted to the hospital or receives care in a nursing home. Here, I'm going to focus primarily on home health aides, who help individuals with ADLs and IADLs at home. According to the Bureau of Labor Statistics' Standard Occupational Classification system,[3] home health aides may conduct certain clinical tasks under the supervision of a licensed professional, such as monitoring vital signs, performing range-of-motion exercises, or administering medications, but the extent of these clinical responsibilities varies by state and setting according to nurse delegation rules, provider policies, and norms of practice. With almost 2.6 million workers,[4] home health aides and personal care aides who provide care at home comprise the largest segment of the direct care workforce, which is unsurprising given the magnitude of individuals in the United States requiring assistance at home as a result of physical, cognitive, developmental, and behavioral conditions. For patients with limited caregiving networks or for those with complex care needs (both of which described my family), the reliance on home care workers is an *absolute lifeline*.

What Do Direct Care Workers Do?

Direct care workers of all kinds have historically been inaccurately referred to as unskilled, in addition to being undervalued and undercompensated. Undoubtedly, this work requires considerable technical skill, especially when working with patients with complicated conditions, in addition to incredible physical and emotional strength. During the entire time we worked with home health aides, my dad required "full assist," meaning that he needed help with all activities of daily living. As a result, the amount of physical and emotional energy our aides put into their caregiving was significant, and I depended fully on them to serve as my eyes and ears when I was at work and to look out for signs of infection or other adverse events so that we could prevent unnecessary trips to the hospital and address problems before they got out of control.

I'm often asked what tasks home health aides do, and some variation of the question, *Is it really worth it to secure the assistance of a home health aide?* Below, I highlight many of the routine tasks our home health aides completed weekly to give you a broad sense of the scope of the help you and your loved one might receive. For those of you who are current caregivers, take note of any of these activities with which you might need assistance.

Examples of Assistance Provided by Home Health Aides

- Monitoring vital signs (blood pressure, oxygen saturation, pulse, and temperature)
- Meal preparation and feeding
- Caring for catheters (including cleaning, changing collection bags, and checking for signs of infection)
- Assistance with oral medications
- Transferring the patient from bed to wheelchair, wheelchair to standing, and wheelchair to car
- Assistance with toileting (either in the bathroom or in bed via a bedpan or diapers)
- Assistance with bathing (either in the bathroom or via a bed bath)
- Pressure ulcer prevention (rolling the patient from side to side in bed, strategically placing pillows to relieve pressure)
- Wound care
- Assistance with physical and occupational therapy exercises
- Assistance with walking
- Companionship

The workdays for our aides were always intense, but more so when we had medical appointments scheduled, which meant they assisted my dad in and out of my brother's car and, often, transferred him from his wheelchair to an exam table. The days were even more difficult when he was having a Lewy body disease fluctuation. As it often is for home health aides working with patients with neurodegenerative diseases or severe cognitive impairment, the daily work was exponentially more challenging when my dad's disconnection from our reality meant he couldn't safely partner with the aides to accomplish tasks like taking his medications.

The responsibilities of home care workers are physically and emotionally demanding. Just as the burden among family caregivers is well documented, the burden experienced by direct care workers is vast and deserves equal attention. Home health aides are increasingly providing complex care, and tasks that require intimate or weight-bearing assistance can cause stress, fear, or agitation for workers and families. In this context, it is not surprising that the direct care workforce has some of the highest rates of occupational injury in the United States.[5] Such injuries lead to potential job loss and financial hardship. Moreover, since the support provided by direct care workers requires intimate physical assistance, workers are unable to observe social distancing practices that would otherwise protect them against infectious disease. This reality was significantly amplified during the height of the COVID-19 pandemic.

In addition to these responsibilities, I look back and think about the invisible work our aides did in caring for my dad emotionally. In some ways, this emotional work was just as important as all their other responsibilities. Most of them became my dad's close friends, and several eventually looked toward him as a son would to a father. The aides would delight in hearing my dad's stories of his life, his time in the army, his loves and losses, and the music industry. They would share their own lives and seek counsel during their ups and downs of young adulthood. My dad's shoulder was open to them, just as it had been for me. They would watch movies together, several took piano lessons from my dad in exchange for his own lessons in their native language, and almost all eventually came to *care* deeply for the man they were taking care of.

In many ways, I watched as our group of home health aides became an ad hoc multigenerational family system for my dad. As with many families in the United States, the infusion of home health aides into our daily life became a new model for family and caregiving. Undoubtedly, in the absence of a large family network and friends of his who were still alive or physically capable of visiting, and particularly given my mom's absence from the home they had shared for nearly fifty years, these aides became a significant part of my dad's social support system. The emotional connectedness that naturally emerged between them and my dad was ultimately a gift, but also added a level of intensity to the work, which increased as my dad got closer to death.

Certainly, not all relationships among patients, family caregivers, and home health aides are warm. There was undeniably great variation in the emotional tone among my dad, me, and the nine home health aides who rotated with us over six years. Bringing a home health aide into your home can be complex. Differing opinions about what constitutes appropriate care for the patient can emerge. The home health aide can get caught in the midst of complicated family dynamics. You may find that you and the aide are in full agreement about care-related tasks but clash interpersonally. One caregiver in clinic shared feeling like he relied significantly on a home health aide whom he *needed* but did not *want* in his home. Another caregiver shared with me feeling like her efforts to care for her husband were judged by their home health aide to be inadequate. Yet another shared that the aide she hired to care for her wife expressed homophobic beliefs. My guess is that for many of you who have already enlisted the assistance of home health aides, you've had your own uniquely challenging experiences (though hopefully in addition to good ones).

Ultimately what will be important for you as you integrate a home health aide or other direct care worker onto your team is to keep an open flow of communication. If there are disagreements between you and the aide about the care being provided, address these immediately. If you have disagreements about topics that are unrelated to caregiving, see if you feel comfortable talking through them as soon as possible. You may find that having a monthly "check-in" conversation with them may be helpful. Such conversations might include a discussion of expectations of the aide's role, including hours of duty and tasks to be accomplished, and space for you and the aide to share what's going well and concerns you each may have. Regularly engaging in these discussions can help to normalize an exchange of opinions and set the stage for a more productive dialogue should problems emerge down the line. Ultimately, the healthiest and most proactive relationships between patients, caregivers, and direct care workers are those where each member of the triad can express how they feel about the care, and you can model this type of relationship right from the start.

Employing Direct Care Workers

Most caregivers are shocked to learn that common private insurance carriers, such as Blue Cross or Aetna, do not typically provide coverage for home healthcare. Through this lens, in addition to all the factors discussed in Chapter 4, the limited long-term care resources offered through insurance companies is another form of ageism, another way in which our healthcare system works against those it claims to serve. Nonetheless, there are various routes to facilitating the placement of a direct care worker in your home, and I explore the most common ones below.

Private Pay

The simplest—albeit most expensive—way to hire a home health aide is through a private pay agency, that is, one that does not contract with Medicaid. Payment for aides through these agencies is out of pocket. The cost per hour ranges across agencies, but you can expect to pay between twenty and thirty dollars an hour. If your loved one has taken out a long-term care insurance policy, this policy can be used to pay for these hours. These policies can have profound financial benefits for your family down the line, and I encourage you to take some time right now to explore whether you are in the position to take out such a policy. We were incredibly fortunate that my dad had bought a long-term care policy when he was in his sixties and we used this initially to pay for his home healthcare.

Through a local agency we began by hiring an aide for eight hours a day, five days a week, thinking that we would be able to handle my dad's needs during the remaining time, but soon realized how difficult the physical work of caregiving was. My dad came home from the hospital with no muscle mass, no ability to sit or stand on his own or even hold a cup or feed himself; everything had to be done for him until he regained his strength. We needed more care and soon hired an additional aide to cover the weekends, spending most daytime hours on Saturdays and Sundays with us. We paid twenty-two dollars an hour for care at that time, and from January 2014 to August of that year, we watched as the long-term care policy started to run low.

Despite the cost, there are many benefits of working with agencies like the one we used, including the fact that they provided training to the aides in basic nursing tasks, had a robust rotation of staff to cover shifts if one called out sick or for another reason could not work on a certain day, and ensured that the aides were up-to-date on their vaccinations (e.g., annual flu shots). There was also flexibility in terms of the range of tasks these aides could complete, including taking vital signs and administering oral medications. It also seemed that most of the aides who came to us via an agency appeared to have a skill set that was closer to that of a registered nurse. Our responsibilities in training or supervising them were limited and included providing education about my dad's unique care needs. The downsides of using such agencies include regulations around the minimum number of hours home health aides can be hired, meaning that even the shortest shift is ultimately expensive. There was also an unspoken limitation that was always distressing to me: the reality that the aides who gave their time and energy were certainly not seeing all the pay that the agency acquired from us.

Medicare

In addition to the lack of home healthcare coverage through most private insurance plans, you may be surprised to learn that there is very little coverage through Medicare for home care. Specifically, Medicare Part A (hospital insurance) and Medicare Part B (medical insurance) together cover part-time or intermittent skilled nursing care, that is, skilled nursing care that is needed less than seven days each week or less than eight hours each day over a period of twenty-one days or less. Medicare also covers part-time or intermittent home healthcare, but the latter is only available if your care partner is also receiving skilled nursing care at the same time. In my dad's case, we were able to use his Medicare plan to cover part of the cost of his long-term stays in nursing facilities, as well as the cost of skilled nursing care and physical and occupational therapy sessions that were prescribed by a physician each time my dad was discharged from the hospital to home. Each of these services was time limited and rarely in place for more than two weeks. Both my mom and I were shocked to learn that Medicare does *not* cover twelve- or twenty-four-hour-a-day care at your home, or personal care with activities of daily living like bathing, dressing, or using the bathroom, when this is the only care needed. As was the case for us and so many other families, it is unlikely that you will be able to rely on Medicare to implement and pay for home healthcare.

Medicaid

Unlike Medicare, coverage for home health aides under Medicaid is possible but requires that the care recipient qualify for Medicaid. Like many older adults in the United States, my dad fell into a gray zone financially for many years. He earned too much money through his pension and Social Security checks to qualify for Medicaid, but he earned too little to pay all his bills. When my mom was alive, her income from performances supplemented these checks so that they could live reasonably comfortably, but after her death, we were in the red. My income as a junior faculty member was not large enough to support us both *and* his care needs, and neither was my brother's, who had just become a father himself. The only way that we could pay for care would be to somehow get my dad onto Medicaid, but to qualify, one's household income cannot exceed 138 percent of the federal poverty limit, based on household size, though this amount fluctuates slightly by state. This poverty level is updated annually by the Census Bureau, and at the time we applied for Medicaid, it was $16,243. Together, his pension and Social Security checks meant that he had an annual income of $42,880, an amount that was well over the Medicaid limit but not nearly enough to live on and pay for medical care, home care, and supplies. Our situation was not unique; Social Security checks are the main source of income for over two-thirds of older Americans, and the sole source for one-third, and rarely if ever are they sufficient to cover the costs of home care.[6]

Back in 2014 I had no idea how to get my dad onto Medicaid. Thankfully, during his first hospitalization after my mom's death, a social worker who was assisting with his discharge suggested I consult with the New York Legal Assistance Group (NYLAG), a civil legal services organization that combats economic, racial, and social injustice by advocating for people experiencing poverty or crisis. Importantly, if you don't know how to begin the process of securing Medicaid coverage for your care partner, speaking with a social worker at the hospital where they receive care is a *great* place to start. You can also search state by state for organizations like NYLAG in all fifty states and territories that can provide you with similar assistance.[7] Through NYLAG, I was paired with a lawyer who walked me through the process and regulations around getting Medicaid coverage for the aged and disabled. What I learned was that under federal law, all states have a way for families to directly pay Medicaid the difference between the patient's monthly income and the Medicaid income limit, thus allowing the patient to qualify for Medicaid. Depending on your state, this difference between your care partner's income and the Medicaid limit that is paid back to Medicaid is called a spend-down, a medically needy program, an excess income program, or a special needs trust.

In early 2015 I completed a Medicaid application for my dad, which required his birth certificate and other identifiers, as well as copies of his pension and Social Security checks, and a breakdown of his medical expenses. This type of task is one of the many reasons why it's helpful that you are the power of attorney for your care partner, so that you can have easy access to their financial documents needed for care-related hurdles like Medicaid applications. The application also included documentation of his disability from his physicians and how funds from Medicaid would be used (that is, to pay for home healthcare). At the same time, I applied to the Center for Disability Rights for an account in the pooled trust and included documentation of this process in our Medicaid application. Funds deposited into the Supplemental Needs Pooled Trust are not counted against the person when applying for Medicaid and can be used for other supplemental needs above and beyond what is covered by Medicaid. Pooled trusts are available across the country by a variety of names, so when you begin to explore your state-specific Medicaid guidelines, it will be important to learn where your funds can be deposited and what the application process might be like.

Once our paperwork was submitted, we were scheduled for a visit from a Medicaid case manager who evaluated our home for safety and the need for equipment, such as grab bars in the shower and wheelchair ramps. A few weeks later, I received word that while the overall application was approved, my request for twelve hours a day of care was denied, and we were approved only for half that time. This was shocking, as my dad's application was supplemented by letters from his physicians documenting his limitations and his requiring "full assist," or help with all activities of daily living. There was no way that six hours a day would be sufficient. It would be dangerous at best. My dad could not get out of bed without an aide helping him and staying in bed for extended periods of time meant bedsores, and bedsores meant infections and bouncing back to the hospital. Translation: *Home health aides equal preventive medicine and cost savings, as one Stage III or higher bedsore costs at least $14,000 to treat.*[8] This was also in the pre-pandemic era when working primarily from home was not an option for me, so there was no way that I could be home half a day, every day, to compensate for when we didn't have an aide.

I had to fight back and appeal the decision, which required my having a Medicaid hearing where I nervously shared why the initial determination was detrimental to my dad's well-being. This step was successful, and in June 2015, two months after my dad's long-term care policy ran out, he was officially enrolled in Medicaid, with a spend-down sent to the Center for Disability Rights Pooled Trust. Moving forward, I would pay some of his medical bills through the trust, and Medicaid would pay for the home health aide, twelve hours a day.

I've heard many caregivers compare their experiences to that of Sisyphus, who in Greek mythology was punished for cheating death by having to roll an immense boulder up a hill only for it to roll down the moment it reached the top.[9] This Medicaid journey was my Sisyphus moment. Each time I thought I had established a solid care plan, I was met with additional barriers. After successfully appealing the initial Medicaid decision, I learned of two additional significant limitations of enlisting the help of home health aides paid directly through Medicaid of which you should be aware going into this process.

First, there are state-by-state regulations about what home health aides contracted through Medicaid can or cannot do. At the time we applied for Medicaid in New York State, home health aides were allowed to assist with personal care tasks, such as bathing, dressing, cooking, cleaning, and grocery shopping, but not nursing tasks such as administering medications. This severely limits the assistance they can provide, especially in the context of patients who are disabled and even bedbound. This posed a significant challenge for us, as my dad was unable to reliably take the small pills prescribed to him. His limited vision and tremulous fingers meant he needed someone's help at 9 a.m., 3 p.m., and 9 p.m. to take his medications on schedule. If an aide couldn't do it, I would need to be home during those times, and that was not feasible if I was going to continue to remain employed.

Second, Medicaid assigns the aide to your family; you have no say in who they are. On a Monday morning in late June 2015, a young woman with a very slight build arrived at our home. She met my dad and immediately told me that she couldn't safely transfer him out of bed to take care of his basic needs. So, while we had finally gotten care covered, it wasn't safe or sufficient.

If you are working to secure Medicaid coverage for your loved one, I want you to keep both of these limitations in mind so that you have realistic expectations before you begin the process.

Self-Directed Medicaid Home Care Services

The above challenges were solved through the Consumer Directed Personal Assistance Program (CDPAP), a New York State Medicaid program. The CDPAP is available in other states by a variety of names, so I encourage you to explore what correlate program is available in your state. The CDPAP allows for the implementation of adequate support that allows a disabled person to live safely and with dignity in their home. The CDPAP is available to patients eligible for Medicaid to, in effect, become the home care agency head and select, train, and direct their own home health aides. By definition, my dad as the recipient of Medicaid was the "Consumer," but since he was unable to manage his home healthcare on his own, I was appointed as the "Consumer Representative." This meant that once my dad was approved for Medicaid and subsequently enrolled in the CDPAP, as the Consumer Representative, it was my job to find the "Consumer Directed Personal Assistants" (aka the home health aides), train them, and place them in shifts. Medicaid still determined the number of hours of care that they would cover and the hourly rate, but everything else was under my control.

Like I did, you can find and hire aides through what is called the "gray market," that is, through websites like Care.com or by word of mouth. You can request a reference letter and documentation of credentials from each aide you interview, or at least ask to speak with one of the families they worked with in the recent past. I found these conversations with other caregivers extremely helpful in determining whether a potential home health aide would be a good fit for our family. If you are currently employing an aide but are interviewing someone new, you might consider having the candidate shadow your current aide and practice one aspect of care. For us, I found having the candidate practice transferring my dad from his bed to his wheelchair would allow us to quickly evaluate their strength, their communication skills, and their approach to patient care. You might also consider asking the candidates about their experience in conducting specific care tasks needed at home, such as taking vital signs or working with catheters.

Once hired, if you are planning on having the aide assist with medications, it will be the Consumer's job, or your job as the Consumer Representative if they are unable, to prepare the medications for the aides to administer. For me, that meant I put my dad's pills out weekly into a pill organizer and provided guidance to the aides as to which pills needed to be given and when.

The benefits of the CDPAP meant that my dad and I had choice over who we employed, which meant that only individuals who were physically strong enough to do the arduous work of "full assist" caregiving were hired. The CDPAP also allows the Consumer Directed Personal Assistant to handle the trifecta of personal care, home health tasks, and skilled nursing tasks. This meant that the aides we hired through the CDPAP could handle my dad's medications and assist with other nursing tasks, like cleaning the opening to his suprapubic catheter and assisting with wound care. While the responsibility on me was greater in terms of the finding, interviewing, hiring, and training the aides, ultimately the flexibility and control it afforded us was well worth it. Additionally, unlike the aides who we had hired from the agency, I felt good knowing that they would be taking home 100 percent of the funds given to them.

Importantly, while I hired home health aides to serve as my dad's Consumer Directed Personal Assistants, it is possible for some family members to serve as Personal Assistants as well. If, for example, my brother had been handling all of my dad's care needs, we could have designated him as the Consumer Directed Personal Assistant and paid him through the CDPAP. This is important to keep in mind if you are *not* the Consumer Representative and if you are able to physically handle your loved one's care needs, as *you* may be able to be paid for your efforts! There are state by state regulations regarding who can serve as a Personal Assistant, such as in New York State, where a spouse of a patient cannot serve as a Personal Assistant. What's important for you to know is that it *is* possible for some family members to be paid by Medicaid for taking on caregiving responsibilities, and you should check what guidelines exist in your state that govern eligibility.

The many steps it took for us to secure a safe and sustainable plan to support my dad's care at home were overwhelming for me. My hope in sharing them is to help prepare you and streamline the steps you take to establish a plan for home healthcare for your loved one. We were incredibly lucky that we lived in a state with one of the more generous Medicaid eligibility rules. Since Medicaid rules—and wait times for approvals—vary by state, it will be important for you to speak to your local Medicaid office or legal assistance organization for more information about what benefits may be available and how you can begin the process.

*   *   *

The involvement of direct care workers is a topic that is often a surprise to caregivers I see in clinic. This may be partly because many of the cancer caregivers who come for support have much shorter caregiving trajectories than I had, characterized by an intense period of caregiving and then either recovery of patient functioning or patient death, limiting the need for assistance from direct care workers or the opportunity to put aides in place. Indeed, the cancer caregiving experience lived by so many of my patients is intense and episodic,[10] and qualitatively different from that of long-haul dementia or other chronic disease caregiving. That said, frequently the possibility of having someone assist with caregiving responsibilities is not even on caregivers' radars, though the benefits of direct care worker involvement are vast.

This was the case for Wesley, who came to me soon after his wife Violet's uterine cancer recurred. Wesley and his wife were both in their early eighties, and neither of them had extended family in the area or friends to whom they felt comfortable delegating caregiving responsibilities. Most of their peers had already had experience with illness and loss, and many of them were either living with adult children or transitioning to assisted living facilities for additional support. Violet and Wesley had prided themselves on being the "youngest old couple" they knew, and up until Violet's cancer diagnosis, they had been fully self-sufficient and enjoying extensive travel and the freedom of retirement.

When Violet was first diagnosed, Wesley found the work of caregiving challenging but manageable. Since he was retired, he could devote all his time to her. He still drove and brought Violet into the city for her weekly appointments, helped her to take her medications, and cooked foods that were palatable to her when she felt sick from the treatments. He shared that this period reminded him in some ways of taking care of Violet during her pregnancies, although the emotional tone of the experience was quite different. Violet was someone who prided herself on being self-sufficient and struggled to accept help, including from her husband. Before she retired, she had had a successful career in law, and was regarded by colleagues as a "fierce litigator." Her journey with cancer forced her to be vulnerable in ways she had never been before, and like many patients, she struggled with feelings of powerlessness, especially in the face of intense symptoms and side effects and an uncertain future. She had also been a caregiver many times throughout her life—to her parents, her children, and even friends—and like many lifelong caregivers, she found giving up control and stepping into the patient role quite challenging. Wesley and Violet often argued about her resistance to accepting help, as she felt like she could handle everything on her own and pushed Wesley away when he tried to help even when she was visibly weak.

In session, I brought up the topic of their hiring a home health aide to assist Violet throughout the week and especially when Wesley was out of the house. Unlike many of the younger caregivers I've supported who were balancing eldercare and childcare and multiple competing responsibilities, in retirement Wesley and Violet had no financial obligations other than taking care of themselves, and they could devote some of their savings to cover the cost of a private pay aide. However, Wesley was resistant to the idea and felt that if his wife needed help, he should be able to do it and that there was no reason to "bring a stranger" into the house.

But a few months later, after Violet fell as she stumbled from the sofa en route to the bathroom one afternoon, I brought up the topic again. At that point, Violet's cancer was not responding well to treatment, and despite her desire to continue to try to "beat it," both knew that she would eventually die from the disease. This time Wesley was more open to the idea of having help, as he recognized the nature of the support he was going to need to give to Violet was changing and would involve more intimate acts, like assisting her with bathing and using the toilet. But when he suggested their hiring an aide, she remained adamantly opposed. She impressed upon him how important her privacy was, and how with whatever time she had left, she did not want it spent with "strangers wiping me." Wesley wanted to honor her wishes and refrained from securing home care.

Ultimately, however, Wesley realized that their rejecting outside help had an adverse impact on their relationship and their well-being. Violet found it emotionally distressing to have her husband help with intimate acts, and Wesley became increasingly frustrated with how difficult each trip to the shower became. As opposed to using these moments as opportunities for connectedness and expression of love, they turned into heated arguments, one of which ended with Wesley yelling and running from the bathroom, something he later regretted.

Just a few months later, Violet transitioned to hospice care. Through that program she was assigned a home health aide who visited several days a week and assisted her with many of the tasks that Wesley had been doing. He shared with me during one of the few sessions we had during that time that the aide's presence allowed him to exhale in a way he hadn't for months, and that Violet allowed herself to be vulnerable and cared for by the home health aide. Wesley regretted not employing an aide sooner and capitalizing on the time they had together when Violet was stronger. He had assumed that involving help earlier on would have detracted from their time together, but he recognized that instead the opposite would have been true.

This sentiment is a common one shared in the clinic. As I did with Wesley, I often introduce the idea of home care workers early on when I meet with caregivers so that they're aware of the possibility of help at home, and steps can be taken to explore options for care long in advance of its being needed. And mission accomplished: The idea of working with a home health aide is now on your radar.

To help keep this idea on your radar and to facilitate a dialogue between you, your care partner, and other family members, in Exercise 7.2 I provide questions that can help guide you and your family in decision-making around home healthcare. None of these decisions are easy, and certainly none occur in a vacuum. Taking some time to think through these on your own and to discuss them with your loved one(s) can be tremendously helpful as you move through your journey as partners in care.

Exercise 7.2: Questions to Facilitate the Implementation of Home Care

- What caregiving responsibilities do you need help with now? Which responsibilities do you think you may need help with in the future?
- Are there any personal care tasks that your care partner does not want you or other family members/friends to take care of?
- What concerns do you and your care partner have about enlisting the help of a home health aide?

- How might you and your care partner benefit from enlisting the help of a home health aide?
- Have you discussed the possibility of enlisting the help of a home health aide with your care partner? Why or why not?

*   *   *

While writing the first draft of this chapter in April 2021, I took a break midway through to walk through Central Park, to take in the spectacular and time-limited visual display of the cherry blossoms and connect to the energy of a city coming back to life after the first wave of the COVID-19 pandemic. I wandered across the park in the direction of the apartment where I grew up, the apartment where my dad spent his last years. I turned off WQXR, which was playing through my earbuds, to allow myself to be fully enveloped by the spring. I was lost in memories as I walked, thinking about Saturday mornings with my dad, and the work that his aides had done each day. I looked around at the many people lying out in the sunshine, at the musicians who were finally able to perform for audiences after a year of pandemic-induced isolation, and a group of children running toward an ice cream truck. In the distance, I saw an older man being pushed in a wheelchair, his head hung low, his shoulders shrugged, his hands clasped. For a moment I imagined it was my dad in that wheelchair, out for some fresh air. A lump formed in my throat and tears came to my eyes. I looked again and was startled to see that the gentleman pushing the wheelchair was one of the aides who worked closely with us for several years, one of the aides on whom many of my reflections in this chapter are based. He walked toward me pushing his patient, not recognizing me behind my N95 mask until I said his name out loud and he stopped. We hadn't seen each other since the day after my dad's death, and the exchange we had in the park was quite brief as he was working and accompanying both his patient and a family member, but it all came rushing back. *Thank you, universe, for this perfectly timed synchronicity.*

We exchanged a brief hello in the park and then I kept walking, eventually finding myself home and back in front of my computer. Shortly after, I received a text from him saying how nice it was to see me and how much he missed my dad. And me. I couldn't think of a more perfect event to happen while writing this, because I realized, too, that I missed him. Not only had he and all the aides taken such good care of my dad but they had also taken such good care of me. They allowed me to live some semblance of a normal life, their presence allowed me to continue to work, and they allowed my dad to engage as fully as possible in life. I realize now, just as I stood by my dad, all our aides stood by my dad, and equally importantly, they stood by me.

CHAPTER 8

Surfing the Waves of Grief

Stairway to Heaven

Artist: Neil Sedaka with Stan Applebaum
and His Orchestra, 1960

Most caregivers think about the death of their loved one at least briefly. Whether that loved one has a very treatable Stage I cancer or early-stage Alzheimer's disease, or a more invasive and deadly inoperable cancer, the thought of death crosses the minds of all caregivers and can deeply impact their emotional experience. However, these thoughts are not always indulged, let alone shared. Frequently in sessions I'll sense significant resistance to talking about death; it is a formidable elephant in the room. And yet, it is often through inviting that elephant in that we develop the capacity to sit with painful emotions and move healthfully through grief. Ultimately, giving space and permission to sit with the idea of death and discuss the many emotions it elicits is incredibly powerful, and freeing. Doing so allows us to learn from death, both before it happens and after.

Metaphors are often helpful in therapy, especially when speaking about difficult emotional experiences like death. And so, when discussing these topics, I often use the metaphor of having your soul amputated. Physically, you may look the same as you did before your care partner died, but a significant part of you is gone. Just as individuals recovering from amputations require care and long periods of rehabilitation, so, too, do you need support to adapt, not only to the loss of your loved one but to the loss of the caregiving role. For many, bereavement is a natural and expected part of the caregiving trajectory, and like everything else I've discussed, some preparation—even if it is just reading this chapter—can be beneficial.

* * *

My dad's death was somewhat shocking to me, not because I was unaware of his fragile state but because he rebounded so many times over the decade before his death that when his body finally stopped working, it took me by surprise. He died in the ICU, after I brought him into the hospital four days prior with what seemed like many of the infections he had had previously, though this time he was thinner and weaker. Before taking him to the hospital I asked what I could do to help him, and he answered by telling me to bring him a pickled herring sandwich. This statement, from the son of a butcher and a lover of all things Jewish, was a great indicator of orientation. He still wanted to live and enjoy the pleasure of eating, but sadly his body was too weak to combat what eventually was an infection that had little to do with his Lewy body disease.

My dad died in the ICU in the morning of February 23, 2019. Thankfully, we had spoken often about what an ideal death would look like long in advance of that ICU stay. From his perspective it meant being free of pain and preferably having it happen while lying in my arms. After my mom's sudden death five years earlier, many of our discussions focused on the eternity of the soul, and we wondered about the possibility of his being held on both sides of the veil by the two women who loved him when he made his transition.

Though perhaps in a different fashion than originally imagined, these goals were met. We couldn't manage at home what was suddenly becoming intense pain from a leg wound that I suspected was a malignancy, but the IV Tylenol he was given in the ICU did the trick. He was comfortable and smiling in the last picture and video I took of us at 8:45 p.m. the night before he died, feeling better than he had in a week. I was looking forward to spending the next morning doing our usual Saturday morning ritual of WQXR and crossword puzzle, but that never happened. Thankfully, I was able to wrap my arms around his shoulders and put my lips to his cheek as he took his last breath.

In the days, weeks, and months that followed, I felt like I was experiencing life through rubber cement. Everything felt blurry, slow, and muted. It felt like a significant portion of my soul had been amputated, and like amputees who perceive pain in the limb that is no longer there, my phantom limb pain was excruciating. I longed so desperately to hear my dad's voice and to look into his bright blue eyes. The weight of the finality and permanence of his absence was crushing. I took several months away from work, as the idea of facing colleagues—let alone my patients—was unbearable. I was going through the motions of my day and on the outside looked as if I was okay, but internally, I felt broken.

What Is Grief?

Many caregivers will ask me to tell them what to expect in terms of grief, how it will feel, and how long it will last. In response, I always emphasize that grief is very personal, and there is no one universal timeline for when it will dissipate. In fact, we cannot and should not expect that as soon as we reach the twelve-month mark, that we will feel completely fine. Certainly, the first year is a year of "firsts," such as first birthdays, anniversaries, Mother's and Father's days, and while after that first year has ended there may be a lessening in the intensity of grief, it doesn't mean a second, third, or even tenth anniversary or other life milestones won't be painful. The wound left by the amputation needs attention and healing, and even when you've begun to adjust to the loss, a scar will always remain. Even if you are moving healthfully through your bereavement journey—meaning that you experience grief but slowly resume engagement in life and the grief does not impair your ability to do so—the pain can be, and often is, felt for many years after.

So, what is grief? *Grief* is a response to loss. It is what you think and feel internally after a loved one dies, and it can include sadness, fear, loneliness, panic, pain, and yearning. It is normal and expected that you will cry, will have difficulty sleeping, lose your appetite, and generally struggle to engage in typical daily life. Conversely, you may show emotional numbness and feel disconnected from the intensity of your sadness, at least initially. You may also have difficulty with memory and attention and concentration, something that has been referred to as "grief brain" or "grief fog." You may be generally unable, at first, to function at the same capacity as you did before the death. The immediate adjustment to the amputation comes with many side effects that require tender attention, patience, and care. It is expected that you will need time to resume engagement in life and that your grief will involve intense emotional pain for at least several months. When you enter bereavement, the period after the death of your loved one during which grief is experienced, it is common to express grief through outward expressions of mourning.

There is an added layer of loss when the person for whom you provided care—for days, weeks, months, and often, years—dies. The death means the end of your caregiving responsibilities. For some of you, this may come with a significant sense of relief; it means being freed from responsibilities that you may not have chosen, and which challenged the carrying forward of other life goals and responsibilities. For others of you, there may be additional grief in losing this role, this part of your identity, the sense of responsibility and necessity and purpose that came with caregiving. Caregiving demands a life orbit around the patient, and therefore, for many long-haul caregivers such as myself, death means a shifting of one's entire existence. This presents complexity for the bereaved caregiver, as caregiving can be both protective against and a risk for maladaptive adjustment to grief. Inevitably, the deaths that are most painful and difficult to process are those of the individuals who are closest to us. For many of you, the person for whom you are (or were or will be) providing care falls into that category, as they are the person around whom your life has orbited, often for many years. Through this lens, the caregiving journey can be looked at as a period in which to prepare for the death of the patient. I certainly had many years of preparation for my dad's death, whereas my mom's death came completely out of the blue and afforded me with no preparation. At the same time, with one's life centered around the patient, the loss is inevitably momentous.

It's important to note that you may feel grief in advance of the actual death of your care partner. That is, you may experience *anticipatory grief*, which includes emotions, thoughts, and behaviors that occur in response to an impending loss.[1] Anticipatory grief is experienced by nearly 40 percent of caregivers and is a normal part of the grief continuum.[2] At the same time, you may also experience very real losses in advance of the death.[3] These pre-death losses are varied and can include: a loss of roles, such as a loss of a sense of a romantic partnership when one partner is sick and unable to participate fully in the partnership; a loss of the patient's capacity to communicate;

a loss of various physical capacities in the patient; and a loss of hope for future experiences with the patient.

A question I frequently hear in clinic is "What can I do to make this grieving process go faster?" My unsatisfying answer is that there is no fast-forward button, and for good reason. Experiencing grief is healthy and adaptive; we need to feel the pain of separation. Our brain needs time to adjust to the amputation, and while the phantom limb pain can be intense, it's important to feel. The instinct to want to avoid pain—to avoid thoughts about death and dying and just move on—is unhelpful and will eventually serve to prolong the process. Like with all bright pink elephants, trying not to think about grief inevitably leads to some intensifying of thoughts about death. In fact, neuro-imaging studies have found that when we try not to think about death, our brain needs to monitor for cues of grief, meaning, actively trying not to think about death inevitably leads us to think about it more![4]

As opposed to avoiding these thoughts, a more helpful approach is to allow them in. I liken thoughts about death to feeling the waves of a freezing-cold ocean on a sunny early summer day. If you allow them to come up and touch your toes, you'll be startled at first by how uncomfortable it is, but after a few waves, the intensity diminishes. You can adjust to the water and walk in a little farther, eventually allowing your feet to be enveloped completely in the sea. Inevitably, the waves will recede, and you'll feel the dry warm sand under your toes. The initial feelings associated with grief are uncomfortable. They are painful. They are sharp like ice-cold water on your toes. But if instead of trying to get rid of them, the moment you feel them fully, you take a deep diaphragmatic breath in through your nose and out through your mouth, you'll feel yourself adapting and better able to sit with the feelings. Doing this will put you directly in touch with pain, but with it, growth and healing. Indeed, the only way out is through.

Trajectories of Grief

Despite what sometimes can look similar on the outside, the healthy grieving process is different from depression. For example, those who are depressed often have negative thoughts about themselves (such as, *I am unworthy of love*), the world (*No one values me*), and the future (*Things will never get better*). These individuals struggle to connect to any positive feelings. On the other hand, despite intense sadness, the bereaved who are not depressed are often able to connect, even if briefly, to positive feelings when thinking about the past, such as smiling or laughing when reflecting on a happy memory of the person who died.[5]

Some bereaved caregivers, however, experience grief that becomes impairing and even dangerous. In addition to intense yearning and preoccupation with thoughts or memories of a care partner, some caregivers experience disabling symptoms, including a dramatic sense of disbelief about the death, feeling that life is meaningless as a result of the death, and difficulty reintegrating into one's relationships and activities after the death. For a small number of caregivers, these symptoms can persist over a year after the death of a care partner and contribute to significant mental health concerns. I want to make it clear that it *is* healthy and expected that you will experience some of these symptoms. But the intensity and range of these symptoms, and their debilitating nature, prevents some caregivers from reengaging in life, leading to further isolation and disconnection.

Research has identified risk factors for such mental health concerns in bereavement.[6] These include prior experiences of loss, trauma, or mental health challenges; having a relationship with the person who died that was characterized by a high level of dependency; poor patient quality of life toward the end of life; perceiving the death as traumatic or unexpected; experiencing stressful and even traumatic medical events during caregiving; and in bereavement, experiencing a high level of regret, shame, or guilt, or struggling to maintain a sense of meaning and purpose.

Certainly, caregiving can be traumatic. It can be traumatic to witness scary medical events like seizures or delirium; it can be traumatic to ride in an ambulance and not know if your loved one will be alive by the time you arrive at the hospital; and it can be traumatic to witness a loved one decline and eventually die, even if the death is expected. These traumatic experiences, these caregiving-related traumas, can contribute to mental health challenges in bereavement.

While it is impossible to avoid all these potential risk factors, receiving support and mental health care during your caregiving journey can protect your future mental health and overall well-being. A mental health professional can help identify risk factors for, and signs of, challenges in bereavement and help you to receive care that is targeted to your specific needs.

In Exercise 8.1, I provide a list of questions that you can use to explore the intensity of your grief. Each one of the concerns listed will likely occur for everyone who is bereaved, at least once. My point in including them, therefore, is not to pathologize your experience of grief. Grief is normal, and all the feelings listed are feelings that most bereaved caregivers experience. However, these questions get at the intensity of symptoms and how impairing they can be for some caregivers. These questions are particularly important to ask yourself if it has been over a year since your care partner died, and you find yourself feeling stuck in your grief. If you answer *yes* to many of these questions, it may be particularly beneficial for you to connect with a mental health professional for further evaluation. In Chapter

10, I discuss ways in which you can find mental health care and what types of support may be most helpful.

Exercise 8.1: Assessment for Mental Health Concerns in Bereavement[7]

- Do you experience intense yearning and longing for your loved one on most days?
- Are you preoccupied with thoughts or memories of your loved one or with the circumstances of their death?
- On most days, do you feel like a part of yourself has died since your loved one's death?
- Even though many months have gone by, on most days are you in disbelief that the death occurred?
- Do you avoid reminders of the person who died?
- On most days, are you in intense emotional pain related to the death?
- Have you had difficulty on most days reintegrating into relationships and activities? Planning for the future?
- Do you feel like life is now meaningless?
- Do you feel intense loneliness on most days because of the death?

Regardless of whether you seek mental health care or not, there are certainly some things that you can do to help yourself cope with grief. First, the benefits of community support and communal grief practices can be profound. For some of you, this community and communal grief practice may go hand-in-hand with religious practice. But you certainly don't need to belong to a religious community to receive support. If you have a network of family and friends, however big or small, making a point to spend time with others and be supported by those who care about you can be beneficial. Even if it's just with one trusted friend, any ways in which you can lean on others emotionally can help you to adapt to the loss. This is one of the reasons why having funerals and memorial services can be so meaningful: They serve the dual purpose of honoring the person who died and bringing together mourners to support one another in their waves of grief.

In addition to having the support of others, emotional expression is an important tool in coping with loss. By this I mean that in bereavement, expressing the range of intense negative emotions you may feel—whether that is done publicly or privately—can help to promote your adjustment to the loss. In fact, I have shared with friends that after each of my parents died, one of the facets of Judaism that I appreciated the most is the way the expression of grief is honored, encouraged, and protected by Jewish rituals. The practice of *sitting shiva* refers to a period when those who suffer the loss remain at home and are visited daily by family and friends who share in the experience of mourning. The purpose of shiva is to provide a time for spiritual and emotional healing, a safe container for grief. Sitting shiva normalized the expression of my grief, and in many ways gave me permission to fully indulge my emotional experience. In traditional Jewish practice, it is anticipated that the bereaved will not leave the home or participate in typical daily activities during the first week after the death, and the first month of mourning is demarcated as an intense and expected period of grief. Children who mourn the loss of a parent do so formally for one year. Grief is normalized. It is accepted that it exists and accompanies the bereaved as they go through the days, weeks, months, and even years after the death.

While I wasn't raised religiously in an Orthodox Jewish fashion, after my mom died I learned the mourner's Kaddish, a prayer that is written in Aramaic and which is traditionally recited in memory of the dead, although it makes no mention of death. Each day I would sit next to my dad and hold his hand, and we would recite the prayer together. Neither of us knew what the words meant, but that didn't matter. Each time we would speak them, our eyes would well up with tears and allow for a much-needed emotional release. The daily ritual gave us a structure for our grief, a place to hold our emotions. A daily check of our grief barometer, per se. Over time we noticed that we were able to get through more and more of the prayer without breaking down, and as the months went by, we noticed that on some days, our urge to cry had dissipated. This shift for us both was accompanied by a new type of sadness, a feeling of disconnection in some way from my mom, fueled by a lessening in the intensity of grief. Our grief connected us to her.

This is a feeling shared by many caregivers, and perhaps is something you have felt as well. Despite how painful this period can be, at some point in sessions many bereaved caregivers express some variation of the following thought: *I don't want the grief to end, because it connects me to [my loved one].* In many ways, grief is the form love takes when someone dies.[8] When we grieve—when we express our pain—we are expressing our love for and attachment to the person who has died. For some, there can be comfort in thinking about the intensity of one's grief as a reflection of love for the person who just died. With this association, however, there is often the downstream thought that if one were to stop grieving, then the connection with the deceased would end. Inevitably, this is where much of my therapeutic work with the bereaved occurs, through helping caregivers to develop new ways to feel connected to their loved one, to maintain the attachment despite the loss and the eventual mitigation of grief.

For many, this is accomplished through rituals, such as creating a space at home with pictures and mementos of the person who died and spending time regularly deep in thought in that space or writing letters each week to the person who died to share thoughts that would have traditionally been expressed in person. For others, these rituals include wearing clothing or jewelry of the person who died or engaging in activities that they had once treasured. The rituals we choose are personal and unique, but what they share is the capacity to help us maintain our sense of connectedness to our loved one who has died, to channel our enduring love for that person.

Each of your experiences of grief—from the death of pets to the death of grandparents, parents, partners, children, siblings, and friends, to colleagues and neighbors—can shape your subsequent experiences. You can learn from past losses about what was helpful and what you could have done differently to cope more effectively. You may also find that earlier experiences of loss may engender within you the capacity to tolerate subsequent grief. For example, my crying each night onto a stuffed toy given to me by the nanny who helped take care of me for the first nine years of my life until she died was my childhood version of saying the Kaddish, so to speak. Without guidance or knowledge of what constituted a healthy grieving process, my nine-year-old self created a daily ritual that allowed my intense sadness to be fully felt and expressed.

If you have already suffered a loss, take a moment and think about the ways in which you expressed your grief, or conversely, efforts you made to hold your grief in. Any ways in which you can allow yourselves to fully ride the waves of grief will not only promote adjustment to the loss but will help to prepare you for any future losses you may experience.

* * *

In September of 2019 I began working with Gary, a forty-eight-year-old widower and single father who was taking care of his nineteen-year-old son, Louis, who had osteosarcoma, a cancer of the bones that is sadly common among children and adolescents. Gary's wife had died of metastatic breast cancer when Louis was just two years old and their daughter, Pauline, was six. After his wife's death, which occurred while she was in the hospital and Gary was home tending to the children, he put all his energy into parenting and doing his best to ensure that his children felt loved and supported. He recounted in our first session never taking time to fully grieve his wife's death. "I never had that luxury," he said.

When we met, Gary shared how painful it was for him to witness his son's health decline and that seeing him weak and bedbound in the hospital was not only intensely sad but reminded him of how his wife looked shortly before she died. Gary was prognostically aware; he understood that his son's cancer could not be cured and would likely kill him, and that the goal of care was moving toward minimizing symptoms and promoting quality of life.

In April of 2020, Louis was admitted to the hospital after spiking a fever. This time, however, Gary was unable to visit. He contracted COVID-19 and isolated himself at home, devastated to miss any moments with his son but aware that exposing his son to COVID-19 would be dangerous. In the early days of the pandemic and without a vaccine in his system, Gary experienced significant symptoms, none of which required his own hospitalization but all of which made leaving his bed, let alone his home, impossible at first. Louis died in the hospital while Gary was home sleeping.

Gary had taken care of Louis every day of his life up until this hospitalization, but when we met a month after Louis's death, he shared feeling like none of that mattered. He had piercing regret at not having been present for his son's death and guilt for what he felt was his letting his son down. After that session, Gary didn't return to see me. I made several attempts to schedule sessions with him, but my calls went unreturned.

I was surprised a year later when Gary reached out and asked if he could return to my care. When he did, he described feeling overpowered by his grief during the intervening months and overwhelmed by images of his son dying. He would spend hours daydreaming about what it was like for his son to take his last breath, and on more nights than not, these daydreams became nightmares that prevented him from sleeping. He continued to punish himself for contracting COVID-19 and for not being in the hospital with Louis during his last days and at the time of his death. He couldn't focus on work and pushed well-meaning friends, and his daughter, Pauline, away when they tried to offer him support. He oscillated between feeling completely emotionally numb and feeling intense sadness when thinking about his son's death, sometimes not believing that it had happened and at other times angrily yelling at the universe about the unfairness of it all. He spent hours replaying the few voice messages from Louis that he had saved, desperate to hear his son's voice and to feel his presence. After several months of isolating himself at home, at his daughter's and friends' urging, he reached out to his primary care physician, who started him on an antidepressant. The medication helped Gary to sleep and regain energy and motivation, and likely contributed to his openness to coming back to see me.

When Gary returned to my care, our work focused initially on the complicated feelings of guilt and regret he felt about missed opportunities for connection with his son during his last weeks of life and the ruminative thoughts that he kept replaying about events in the past. He was desperate to receive forgiveness but knew that he would ultimately need to be the one to grant it. Our sessions helped him to accept the limitations he faced and to acknowledge—and even express pride in—how he had parented Louis and Pauline throughout their lives since their mother's death. We also discussed who Louis was as a young man, the values he held and the hopes that he had. Through reflecting on Louis's values, Gary was able to connect to how Louis would want him to live his life now and ways in which how he chose to live life moving forward would be a means to honor and carry forward Louis's legacy. Through these sessions, Gary realized that he had withdrawn from his relationship with Pauline, in part because he feared letting her down in some significant way, the way he perceived that he had let down his son. It took several more months of our working together before Gary was able to release himself from a vicious cycle of rumination and guilt and allow himself to connect to more pure feelings of sadness. While intensely painful, allowing himself to vulnerably express deep sadness was a necessary step in helping him to eventually adjust to such a catastrophic loss.

Parents like Gary contend with multiple challenges, including what has been termed "off-time" loss,[9] as a child dying does not match what we expect in a typical life trajectory. Parents who lose a child to illness not only experience the devastating pain of their child's life ending prematurely but also the loss of the caregiver role, both as a caregiver when the child was ill and as that child's caregiver more broadly in life.[10] For all these reasons, bereaved parents often experience a deep sense of lost possibilities and a disconnection from their sense of identity.[11] If you suffer the loss of a child, you may find that connecting with other bereaved parents can help you to feel less alone, as will the support of a mental health professional, who can help you to cope with the unique challenges of this type of loss.

How Can I Prepare for Death?

I don't think we can ever be fully prepared for the impact death will have on our lives. However, if your care partner is living with a life-limiting illness, there are ways in which you can begin to prepare yourself for their eventual death, and perhaps not surprisingly, these center around communication. Like all difficult topics, the more you can discuss your fears about death—with your care partner, friends, family, a therapist—the more capable you will feel of facing that eventual death. While inevitably many of the thoughts and fears you have may be rational (such as, "It's going to be excruciatingly painful when my dad dies"), you'll likely have other potentially unhelpful thoughts. For example, I've frequently heard some version of the thought, "I will never feel happiness after they die." Opening a discussion with your care partner about your fears and your ability to cope with loss can give you both the opportunity to share your feelings and even to problem-solve together about facing this ultimate limitation. Talking about death won't make death come sooner (this is a common and unhelpful association I hear), but it can help you to feel a little more prepared.

Since you may not have the guidance of a mental health professional to support you in having these types of discussions, in Exercise 8.2 I've provided some food-for-thought questions for you to think through. These questions can help you clarify the concerns you may have, barriers that may be holding you back from addressing certain topics, and goals for eventually having these discussions. As you begin to answer these questions, it can be helpful to write out some of your thoughts or better yet, share them with a trusted friend. Taking time to practice speaking your fears out loud in advance of doing so with your care partner can help you to feel more confident in having these conversations.

Exercise 8.2: Questions to Guide Discussions about Death

- When you think about your care partner's death, what are your biggest fears? Have you spoken about these fears with them? With friends, other family members, or a therapist? Why or why not?
- When you think about your care partner's death, are there any logistic concerns that come to mind? If so, is there anything you can do now to prepare?
- What are some of the benefits you could imagine deriving from discussing death with your care partner?
- If you have already discussed your feelings about death with your care partner, what was helpful/unhelpful about that conversation?
- Is there a specific question or concern or thought related to death that you would like to share with your care partner but haven't yet? If so, what is holding you back?

It's normal to have concerns about opening these conversations, including fears that having them in the first place may be harmful in some way to your loved one. While you may be ready to discuss the emotional side of death, your care partner may not be. They may be grappling with their own fears of death and worries about the impact of their death on you. This is where some of the communication techniques I discussed in Chapter 5 can come in handy, to help both you and your care partner navigate this delicate moment. For example, agenda setting can help you to frame the conversation you want to have. You might say something like:

> Mom, it was really hard to hear what the doctor said, about there not being any more treatments available to prevent your cancer from spreading. Would it be possible to talk about the future? I have a lot of fears about you not being here, and I think talking about them might be helpful. Can we talk about what this might be like?

Part of what you're doing here when setting the agenda is also having a consent conversation, that is, asking your loved one if it would be okay to talk about death. If their answer is no, that's okay. It might not be no forever. Remember, when you open this discussion, you may be in a different place emotionally than your loved one. They may need some time to open themselves up to this type of conversation. As with all advance care planning discussions, opening these conversations about death can be quite challenging, so having a plan for how to begin them can be incredibly helpful. Practicing setting the agenda out loud in advance of the actual conversation can help you to feel more confident when you do finally have it.

Giving space for difficult emotions is one benefit of talking about death, but another is that the death of a loved one rarely happens in a vacuum and instead is associated with many other life changes and logistic challenges. For example, many caregivers have financial concerns associated with death, such as concerns about how to pay for funerals and burials and how to pay the bills after a loved one's income is no longer available. Others have concerns about how to navigate complicated family dynamics, or the division of belongings or property. Taking time to discuss these concerns will allow you to problem-solve and plan. Doing so won't make the death any less sad, but it will ultimately address some of the anxiety you may be feeling about the downstream logistic impact of death.

I'm often asked, "When is the best time for me to talk to my loved one about my concerns? When is it time to speak about death?" My answer is usually, "Now." It is rarely too early to discuss death, even if death is not likely imminent. In fact, I have yet to hear from a caregiver that opening this conversation was harmful to their relationship with their care partner or that they regretted bringing it up. It is the opposite—intense regret in bereavement over not having had an open dialogue about death—that I hear more often. Opening these conversations can feel scary and overwhelming, but inevitably once you do you will take an exhale.

These conversations frequently go hand-in-hand with the advance care planning discussions I covered in Chapter 5, where the focus is on your loved one's goals of care and ways in which you, as the healthcare proxy, can help to carry those out. Here, however, I'm encouraging you to speak with your loved one about the emotional side of death, their thoughts and feelings, and your thoughts and feelings. Ultimately, inviting death into your discussions allows for vulnerability and intimacy, and over time fosters connectedness between you and your care partner. Having had these conversations, in bereavement you will be able to feel proud and grateful for your initiating them. You'll still feel sadness, but you likely will feel less regret. In fact, when I reflect upon the past decade of my work, one of the most important interventions I have enacted in sessions is encouraging caregivers to have these conversations early, at times when their loved ones are able to engage meaningfully in them. I frame this as preventive medicine for both patients and caregivers; these conversations are a powerful tool to help patients cultivate peace and acceptance of death and for caregivers to buffer mental health challenges in bereavement.

*   *   *

The ability to take time away from work in bereavement is a concern brought up by almost every bereaved caregiver I've worked with. The requirement for many working caregivers to return to work soon after the death of their loved one is a significant challenge. Indeed, like the ability to take time off from work to accommodate caregiving responsibilities, the experience of caregivers in bereavement is very much impacted by both public policy and employer-specific regulations around paid and unpaid leave. Frequently, caregivers will discuss their efforts to plan how much time to take off from work during caregiving, while balancing what they know will be needed time off after their loved one's death. The trend is usually the same: saving days off now, so that they can be taken later. The problem with this trend, of course, is it limits time caregivers may take while their loved ones are still here. Certainly, time will be needed when caregivers enter bereavement, but having to choose between time with a loved one alive and time to tend to grief is a terrible decision to have to make.

I've seen a variety of responses from employers around allowance for time off during bereavement. These have ranged from "three days, period, no questions asked" for one patient who worked at a small nonprofit, to "take as much [paid] time as you need, just let us know when you'd like to return" for a patient who worked for a large tech company. There is no clear, universal policy and no clear, universally best option. We are all wired differently. For some, an immediate return to work is not just necessary but a welcome distraction. For others, including myself, returning to work so quickly was just unthinkable. Of course, my line of work isn't neutral, and so that, too, shaped the risks and benefits of my returning quickly. As does the need for income. A handful of caregivers in the clinic were not concerned about the financial repercussions of time away and could take up to six months off from work unpaid without concern. For others, the possibility of losing just a few days' worth of pay was devastating. So, there is certainly no one-size-fits-all plan for returning to work in bereavement. However, we certainly need policies that allow for all bereaved caregivers to have their unique needs met.

If you are a caregiver in the United States, the extent of bereavement leave granted to you will be determined by both state and employer policies. As of 2023, these policies typically range from three to five days of guaranteed time off for employees who suffer the loss of a spouse, domestic partner, parent, child, or sibling. However, since there are state-by-state policies regarding the specific amount of time granted and additional stipulations based on your employer's discretion, it will be important for you to check with a representative from your employer's HR department about what may be available to you.

Any of you who have already suffered the loss of someone close to you knows that three to five days is not nearly enough time to cope with a deeply life-altering loss, which means that if this is your employer's policy, you may need to supplement these days in other ways. This was something I did after each of my parents' deaths, though in different ways. After my mom's death, the offer of three days seemed almost comical given the shock, trauma, and enormity of all that I was facing. However, I was able to extend my time away using FMLA. If you are taking care of someone else at the time of your care partner's death, as I was for my dad at the time of my mom's death, you can do so by using the Family Medical Leave Act (FMLA),[12] which, depending on your employer and the state you reside in, may pull first from your bank of sick and vacation days, but can allow you to be out for an extended period of time, without being at risk of losing your job or benefits.

Another option available to you is to go out on medical disability for yourself, that is, to take time away from work due to your own health. If you are suffering from a medical or mental health condition that requires treatment by a medical professional, you are eligible to do so, as long as that healthcare provider can document the condition for which you are being treated and which would, if left untreated, prevent you from working. After my dad died, I realized that while FMLA was no longer an option for me since I was no longer taking care of him, I was eligible to go out on medical disability. I had been in therapy for years, engaging intensely for treatment of PTSD that resulted from discovering my mom's death, and over the intervening years for the many emotional ups and downs that come with caregiving. I had a medical record documenting this care, my risk for mental illness given the impending death of the person who was my raison d'etre, and what had become a case of very severe insomnia caused and maintained by the multifaceted stress of caregiving. Going out on disability for a psychiatric reason of course can come with risks, including stigma, even in the setting in which I work. But for me, it was the best and most logical option. As it may be for you.

As you think about what options will be available to you in the future, it's important to acknowledge that FMLA and bereavement policies are often limited to biological and legal family members who are the parents, partners, and children of patients. That means that they do not universally apply to many chosen family members, or friends, or extended family members who are just as often intensely involved in caregiving and experience enormous grief but not recognized formally as eligible for bereavement leave. If you fall into a category not recognized by FMLA or your employer's specific bereavement leave policy, it will be even more important for you to think creatively about how you will be able to take time off from work, both now and in bereavement.

If you are currently employed, do you know what your employer's bereavement leave policy is? Do you know if you are eligible to take advantage of FMLA and if so, how much time will be covered and how much income you can earn while out? If you are not eligible for FMLA, is taking time off from work via disability an option? As it was for me, being under the care of a mental health provider during your caregiving journey has the potential to help you down the line to apply for disability. I encourage you to gather data now so that you are as informed and prepared as possible to facilitate time away from work in the future. In fact, many caregivers have found it helpful early on in their caregiving journeys to speak with HR representatives about what options might be available in the future for time away.

Ultimately, there is no one way to prepare fully for the death of someone we love. We can anticipate it and fear it, chew on it in our minds for years and years (twenty-seven years, even), but when it happens, it's different from anything we can imagine. While I don't think that we can ever change that fact, I do feel hopeful that through speaking more openly about death and discussing our most vulnerable and deepest fears, we can receive the support we need and strengthen our capacity to cope with grief. Death is a natural part of life and, often, caregiving, and ultimately it is an event from which we can all learn.

CHAPTER 9

Finding Meaning in Caregiving

The Goin's Great

Artist: Sammy Davis Jr.
Composed by Stan Applebaum, 1969

Taking care of a loved one with a chronic or life-limiting illness rarely feels like a choice, and even in instances when it is, it's a difficult one to make. Once you're in the role, the challenges of caregiving are significant, and the downstream effects on you can be profound. I have yet to meet a caregiver who has not struggled, in some way, with their responsibilities. If you have been a caregiver before or are currently in the role, you have your own variation on the theme of this statement. At the same time, caregiving is an opportunity to connect to what's meaningful to you, to a sense of purpose both in caregiving and in life more generally. It's a chance to improve your relationship to your care partner and to others in your support network; it's a chance to learn new things about yourself and develop strengths you never imagined possible; and it's an opportunity to redefine the goals you have for your life.

When I think about this co-occurrence of suffering and meaning in caregiving, I use the metaphor of a crème brûlée, which happens to be my favorite dessert. I want you to imagine a creamy, pudding-like baked custard with a brittle top of melted sugar that cracks when you gently tap it with a spoon. Crème brûlée is crispy on the outside and creamy on the inside, it's hot and cold all at once. And when you take that first bite, there is a *lot* going on. In many ways, emotionally speaking, caregiving is like a crème brûlée: you can feel sadness, fear, and anxiety, experience trauma and limitations because of caregiving, and at the same time derive love, connectedness, and an enhanced sense of meaning in life. These contradictory feelings can all exist together, a mix of varying flavors and textures. What this means, then, is suffering and meaning are not mutually exclusive; suffering can coexist with the greatest beauty, joy, and strength.

I want to be clear here that I am not talking about avoidance, or the power of positive thinking, or turning lemons to lemonade. I would never discount the suffering that any of you face; that suffering is real and needs validation and expression. I do hope, however, that I can help you begin to connect to the possibility that alongside your challenges, alongside the many ways in which caregiving has made or may make your life more difficult, caregiving can also serve as a mechanism through which you discover meaning, purpose, and growth.

*   *   *

When I began my postdoctoral fellowship in 2010, one of my primary responsibilities was to provide care to patients with advanced, life-limiting cancers using an approach called Meaning-Centered Psychotherapy.[1] My mentor, Dr. William Breitbart, developed Meaning-Centered Psychotherapy in response to what he recognized was a gap in the traditional repertoire of therapeutic interventions. Dr. Breitbart, who is the son of Holocaust survivors, was influenced by the writings of Viktor Frankl. Frankl was a Jewish psychiatrist living in Vienna at the time of World War II. Because he was such a prominent physician in his community, he and his wife and children were granted exit visas to come to the United States and flee the war. Frankl struggled with this decision, as visas were not granted to his extended family. One morning after the war began, he was walking through Vienna and stumbled upon a rock that had a Hebrew inscription on it. He brought it to his father, who was a Talmudic scholar, who said that it looked as if it had come from one of the tablets of the ten commandments, likely from one of the synagogues that had already been destroyed. Frankl asked his father which commandment was inscribed in the rock, to which he replied, "Honor thy father and thy mother." In that moment, Frankl was reminded that his family was a key source of meaning in his life. He realized that he couldn't imagine leaving any of his family members in Vienna, and so he chose to stay. Ultimately, his entire family was sent to the concentration camps, and only he survived.

Before the war, Frankl had already been developing *logotherapy*, that is, therapy that assists individuals to connect to meaning in life. However, his experiences in the concentration camps solidified his ideas. For example, Frankl suggested that there was something about some of the concentration camp prisoners that allowed them to endure the atrocities with which they were continuously faced, that allowed them to be hardy, a little bit more resilient. He identified this "something" as meaning. In discussing this "something," Frankl quotes Nietzsche, who said:

He who has a why to live for can bear with almost any how.[2]

If you have a *why*, a purpose, then the *how*, the day-to-day, can become more bearable. Frankl felt that those individuals in the camps who could remain connected to their *whys*—which for him meant envisioning his beautiful wife as he looked at the sky—were better able to face the challenges around them with strength. Those challenges, he believed, became greater when one was disconnected from their *why*, their purpose. Frankl also recognized that even though everything had been taken away from him—his clothing, food, and medicine, his belongings, his dignity—the one thing the Nazis did not take away was his mind, his ability to choose how to respond to his circumstances, to the extraordinary challenges and limitations around him. Frankl felt that in the face of suffering, humans retained the ability to choose their attitude, to choose how to respond to the limitations they were facing.[3]

Dr. Breitbart realized that these concepts—finding meaning, choosing how one responds to suffering—were powerful ones for patients who were facing life-limiting illnesses. So, he created Meaning-Centered Psychotherapy,[4] a brief therapy to assist patients to connect to a sense of meaning and purpose in life, despite the finiteness of life. Frankl had suggested that whether we have one year, or one month, or one day, or even just one hour to live, that that time is an opportunity to connect to meaning. Meaning-Centered Psychotherapy helps individuals to do just that.

During my first year at Memorial Sloan Kettering, one of my most memorable patients was a fifty-one-year-old man who came to New York from Jamaica to train in landscape design and eventually worked as one of the primary landscape artists at one of the city's botanical gardens. He had been diagnosed at age forty-five with advanced non-small-cell lung cancer, and the cancer had not responded to either first- or second-line treatments. He knew that his cancer would kill him and likely within the next year.

Using the tools of Meaning-Centered Psychotherapy, we discussed his sense of identity, and how while key aspects of his life and activities had changed since his illness, other important elements of his authentic self remained. For example, he had always had a dry sense of humor and was inquisitive, two qualities that were showcased in our sessions. We talked about the concept of legacy, and how we can leave our mark on the world not just by the work we do or the families we create but by our being witnessed by others, by the impression we leave on others. We talked about the ways in which he had impacted his colleagues and friends, and how the lessons he learned from his mother—*What are you waiting for? Use the fine china!*—were lessons he gave to those close to him (since meeting him I have always used the fine china passed down to me, so her legacy is alive through me as well). We talked about what was so meaningful about his work in the gardens, and how he experienced such a sense of connectedness and joy when he had his hands on the earth.

By the fourth session, which focuses on facing limitations, he was dependent on a continuous flow of oxygen from a tank that he carried next to him in a fashionable floral tote. He was no longer physically capable of getting down on his hands and knees and working for hours in the gardens. However, we discussed ways in which he could connect to that part of his gardening work that was so meaningful and special and landed on the benefits of his making window boxes for his apartment. Creating these boxes could connect him to what was at the heart of his work that was so important to him. All these conversations helped to bring him out of his depression. We never once denied the severity of his illness, or the many aspects of his suffering, or the fact that there was a significant change in his ability to walk back to the counseling center room from our first to our seventh and final session. Instead, we acknowledged the potential to connect to a sense of meaning and purpose despite—or alongside of—this very palpable suffering. We acknowledged the full range of flavors and textures of his crème brûlée, including intense sadness, frustration, pride, connectedness with his authentic sense of self, and the capacity for joy when experiencing life through his five senses.

Meaning and Caregiving

As I accompanied this patient and many others on their journeys of connecting to meaning, I realized that the themes discussed in Meaning-Centered Psychotherapy—identity, legacy, choice, responsibility—were extremely relevant to caregivers. It was also clear from the scientific literature published at the time and from the clinical experiences I had under my belt that finding meaning in or through caregiving could help to buffer the enormous burden experienced by so many caregivers. If taking care of a parent, for example, could provide an opportunity to repair a relationship before the parent's death, or connect a caregiver to inner strength they had not previously recognized, then these effects could provide some balance to the distress so often experienced. I also realized that back then in 2011, there were no therapies that framed the caregiving experience as one that could engender a sense of meaning or purpose, or even one that viewed caregiving through the lens of potential benefits. The therapy literature overwhelmingly focused on burden, distress, and challenges, and very little on the possibility for benefit or growth.

This was particularly striking because seminal research on meaning-making came initially from interviews with bereaved caregivers of men with advanced HIV disease.[5] These men had provided care in the era before anti-HIV drugs turned HIV from a death sentence into a chronic and often manageable disease. Their narratives highlighted their experience of co-occurring great suffering and meaning in the context of providing care to their terminally ill loved ones. Not only were they able to sustain positive morale and develop a sense of resilience during caregiving but, as a result, they did better in bereavement because of this established connection to meaning in caregiving and an overall sense of purpose and growth. Meaning seemed to be a life preserver that allowed them to ride a river of deep grief without drowning. Their way of coping was subsequently labeled as meaning-based coping,[6] and that is exactly what is being fostered through Meaning-Centered Psychotherapy.

It's well-documented that humans have the potential to experience positive change following traumatic experiences, such as natural disasters,[7] interpersonal violence,[8] and war.[9] One patient of mine who was a survivor of intimate partner violence had gone on to commit her life to teaching self-defense to thousands of women and empowering others to leave potentially unsafe situations before they became dangerous. Another patient had lost both of his parents when he was seven years old during the attack on the World Trade Center on September 11, 2001. At twenty-eight, he became an attorney and specialized in family law and adoption. He shared with me that his early childhood experience inspired his desire to provide safe and loving homes for other children without parents. While he could never bring his parents back, this work helped to soothe the deep wound caused by their traumatic death and bring a sense of meaning and purpose to his life.

This potential to experience growth and benefit despite—or in response to—the challenges of caregiving is similarly documented.[10] We are extraordinarily resilient; we can face limitations, trauma, and hardship, and at the same time, experience meaning, purpose, and growth. We can enjoy the most delicious of emotional crème brûlées. According to Frankl, our capacity to do this, this drive to make meaning, is like thirst or hunger. It's a basic motivational force. We are driven to connect to meaning in situations that leave us feeling powerless, as is often the case with caregiving. Connecting to meaning can happen through the choices you make, such as how you choose to face the caregiving role. It can happen through your creative endeavors, including how you create your life while taking care of someone else. And it can happen through how you experience life through your five senses, such as gaining a new appreciation for the peace and even transcendence that comes from simply lying quietly in your loved one's arms. You can look at this role as a source of suffering *and* an opportunity for meaning-making and growth. Doing so has great benefits, including decreased depression,[11] lower burden, and improved physical health, quality of life, and coping capacities,[12] as well as increased satisfaction with life, self-knowledge, and personal growth.[13] Your ability to connect to meaning in caregiving can also improve your relationships with your care partners and lead to feelings of satisfaction, reward, and pride.[14] Additionally, connecting to meaning during caregiving can improve your experience of bereavement, as meaning-making is a powerful way to cope with loss.[15]

What we find meaningful in life and caregiving is very personal and unique to us. There is no one definition of meaning, and no right or wrong way to think about this idea. Before you read further, I encourage you to take a moment and consider your answer to the following question:

What does the word *meaning* mean to you?

Meaning-Centered Psychotherapy for Caregivers

My early experiences in delivering Meaning-Centered Psychotherapy to patients facing life-limiting cancers, combined with my growing professional interest in caregiving superimposed upon my new caregiving role, inspired me to adapt this approach into one tailored for caregivers.[16] Through seven sessions, Meaning-Centered Psychotherapy for Caregivers[17] helps caregivers connect—and reconnect—to various sources of meaning in their lives. The purpose of the approach is not to deny the challenges, burden, and distress associated with caregiving but instead to explore how connection to meaning and purpose can exist simultaneously. Meaning-Centered Psychotherapy for Caregivers helps caregivers to take a bite of that crème brûlée and appreciate all the different flavors and textures. The approach focuses on four sources or categories of meaning—called the *historical, attitudinal, creative,* and *experiential*—that can become resources for you both during and after caregiving. As you read through the following descriptions, I want you to begin to think of ways in which your own experiences, in any area of your life, fall into these categories of meaning.

Connecting to Meaning through Legacy

The *historical source of meaning* refers to meaning you can derive from reflecting on the story of your life. You have a past that you did not choose, that you were born into, that was given to you. The elements of your past that have deeply shaped you are what is called your past legacy. This includes components of your upbringing that had a significant impact on who you are, such as the cultural, religious, and spiritual values of your family of origin. Particularly important elements of past legacy for caregivers include previous experiences of providing care or watching parents and grandparents provide care to friends and family members; past experiences of illness or loss; and religious, spiritual, or familial traditions that promoted commitment to the family. In the present, you are living and creating a life that is in many ways in response to your past legacy, the legacy you were given. For example, the way you are living your life right now may reflect elements of your past legacy that you hold dear, as well as elements that were challenging and thus a motivating force for change. This is your current legacy. Your future legacy is the one you will give to others in the future, and includes specific lessons that you teach others directly, the wisdom that you share, as well as the broader impact you have on others, including how others view you as a caregiver. In this way, your caregiving role sets an example for future generations, family members, and friends. The historical source of meaning is the meaning that you can derive through reflecting on your life as having been lived in this historical context of past, present, and future legacy.

When I think about my past legacy, I think about my maternal grandmother, Ida Notov. She was very much a caregiver from a young age, and that part of her identity was carried through her entire life. For decades, she devoted herself to volunteerism, and until her last years of life, volunteered five days a week at various hospitals in the Pittsburgh area, including Western Psychiatric Hospital and Forbes Hospice. She would reach out to the families of patients who had recently died and offer support, often meeting them regularly for months after the patient's death. She was so beloved by these patients and hospitals that in 1988, she was awarded the American Institute for Public Service Jefferson Award in recognition of outstanding public service.

I didn't put it together until long after her death—after my mom's death, in fact, when I was going through boxes of mementos and found several pictures of my grandmother sitting at the bedside of hospice patients. I realized in that moment that she was doing exactly what I was doing professionally, accompanying patients in their last months, days, and hours, often holding the hands of those who were dying without any family by their sides. I now embrace this legacy I've been given and think back to the regular calls I'd have with my grandmother on Saturday afternoons in which she would tell me about the patients she had seen, the volunteer work she had done. It's clear now her legacy is living through the work that I do.

Connecting to Meaning through Choice

Whether or not you choose to become a caregiver, the way you engage in the role, how you face the challenges presented to you through caregiving, that *is* your choice. The *attitudinal source of meaning* refers to meaning that can be derived through reflecting on how you *choose* to face limitations and challenges, which are so prevalent in caregiving. To be clear, this is not about choosing to feel happy in a situation that makes you sad, or about ignoring the difficulties you're facing. Instead, it is about taking an honest look at where you do have agency. Reflecting on how you respond to challenges can itself be challenging, but it can also be incredibly meaningful, especially because of the lack of choice so many of you face in caregiving. Recognizing *how* and to *what extent* you engage in this role may serve as a catalyst for an improved sense of confidence in your capacity to handle the intense work of caregiving. Additionally, highlighting how you choose to face limitations due to caregiving, such as the inability to make advanced plans, interruptions to personal goals and employment, and often a limited amount of time remaining with your care partner, can foster the development of new skills, clarified values, and resilience that will serve you well in every area of your life.

The concept of choice was brought to life most powerfully for me as I witnessed my dad facing the limitations of his illness. Even when he was bedbound and dependent on others for care, he chose to make the most of every day. From writing music, poetry, and children's stories to giving lessons in music theory, engaging in full-body workouts, and reminding me that his hospital bed tray made a great place for a chessboard, he chose to push himself to make the most of his time, despite his profound limitations. He never allowed himself to get bored or feel stagnant and always chose to find joy and a sense of contentment.

When I think about choice, I also think about how the unpredictability of my dad's illness and the daily uncertainty with which I was living often made it impossible to work, let alone plan for events in the future or vacations longer than a day or so. The inevitable emergencies at the worst moments made it challenging to live some semblance of a typical young-adult life. Yet, I never gave up the hope to have small pockets of normalcy, to take a long weekend away in California, a night out at the ballet, or even just a walk in Central Park. For sure, each of these moments was accompanied by anxiety and constant checking of my phone for texts from my dad's aides about his vital signs and any indication of infection, but each time I chose to prioritize a small part of myself that was desperate to continue to live life fully. This, too, is attitude. I didn't want to be defined by caregiving and I didn't want to give up my life. It's also part of why I did not share my caregiving role with more than just my close colleagues. I wanted to be as "normal" as possible at work; to have an entire day in the office without a startling phone call or text was at the time to me a pure gift, and I wanted to be able to fully enjoy that part of my identity when possible. In Meaning-Centered Psychotherapy for Caregivers, we discuss how through reflecting on attitude, you can begin to feel proud of yourself for how you face limitations and losses. Looking back, I certainly feel proud of how I faced so many challenges, and I hope that you will be able to feel this way as well.

Connecting to Meaning through Creative Acts

You are the author of your life. The *creative source of meaning* refers to meaning you can derive from how you put yourself into the world, how you *create* your life. Frankl uses the metaphor of a sculptor who is chiseling away at a large stone. The sculptor knows that something needs to be created but does not know when the deadline is. The stone is a metaphor for your life, and what is chiseled out, your values, what is important to you. The creative source of meaning is the meaning you derive through how you chisel out your unique stone.

You put yourself into the world through the work you do, the causes you devote yourself to, and the relationships you cultivate. Each of these domains takes creativity. Devoting yourself to someone you love is a creative act, because you are putting your energy into that person and into that relationship. If you are someone with artistic talents, the act of creating your art—painting a painting or playing a piece on the piano—can be a source of meaning. Creating your life also means taking *responsibility* for your life—that is, caring for your body, mind, and soul. This includes how you can continue to create your life and live as fully as possible despite the challenges of caregiving.

My caregiving journey underscored the importance of this creative source of meaning and of taking responsibility for my life. There was no way that I could take care of my dad without making sure that I was okay. And that included continuing to engage in therapy, making sure I was sleeping enough (even if at irregular hours and with the help of medications), eating enough, and protecting myself energetically. I learned to honor my true introverted nature, to cherish my alone time, and to limit or cut altogether communication with individuals who drained my energy. My social circle narrowed but became richer. I learned to say *no* to work projects, something none of us are taught to do in graduate school, and I learned to set emotional boundaries to protect myself. All these skills allowed me to recover and take care of my dad and survive what eventually became an ultramarathon of caregiving. And these are the same skills that carried me through the depths of grief since his death.

Engaging in creative acts often requires courage. Just as it takes courage to allow yourself to fall in love again after your heart has been broken, it takes courage to continue to create your life if you are living with an illness like cancer or dementia. As a caregiver, it takes courage to continue to invest fully in a relationship with a care partner that you know will end or will change due to illness.

Here, when I use the word *courage*, I'm reflecting on a powerful definition, that of Rollo May:

> *Courage is not the absence of doubt but the ability to move forward in spite of it.*[18]

Having courage does not mean that you feel confident in the future and confident in yourself. Instead, it means that you are choosing to continue to create and put yourself into the world/relationship/job/art, despite an uncertain future or outcome, despite not feeling confident in the future or yourself.

Caregiving connected me deeply to this way of thinking about courage. Some caregivers find themselves withdrawing emotionally from their loved ones as they get closer to death. They don't necessarily do this purposefully; instead, the distancing happens naturally as their care partner's decline becomes inevitable, as a way to protect themselves from pain. I remember sitting by my dad's hospital bed at home in late January 2019. My sister-in-law was going into labor with my second nephew, and as I was hearing updates about the new Applebaum life coming into this world, in front of me I watched as another was starting to leave. I realized in that moment something that I'd known deep down all along but that was becoming more evident: I had continued to love my dad fully despite knowing our relationship would end, and my love for him kept growing and there was no way for me to stop it. I realized the inherent risk in allowing my heart to remain so open, knowing it would soon be broken into a million pieces. I was terrified of losing my dad *and* terrified of not loving him fully, of missing out on just one moment of that love while it was still here. Back then, I didn't identify the way I loved my dad during his last weeks, days, and hours as courageous, but I certainly do now.

Connecting to Meaning through Experiences

The *experiential source of meaning* refers to the meaning you can derive through connecting to the world through your five senses, and through feelings of love, experiences of beauty, and moments of humor. For example, through a tight hand-hold or hug, you may feel connected through your love for your care partner; you may be transported from present suffering merely through listening to your favorite music or sharing a laugh at a difficult moment; or feel a sense of tranquility through experiencing the beauty of nature, which often serves as a reminder of the continuity of the world and the connectedness of humans to something much bigger. That's the beauty of the experiential. Your five senses can transport you to a different time and place and lead to some of the most magnificent feelings.

The *experiential source of meaning* can be a particularly powerful resource for both patients and caregivers as a patient's health declines and their capacity to engage in life in the manner they once did diminishes. In fact, it is through connecting to the experiential that you can most powerfully assist your loved one to live as fully as possible for as long as possible. For example, often caregivers will share with me their desire to ensure that their care partner can achieve what's on their "bucket list," such as taking a special trip or reaching a certain milestone. But achieving these milestones is often unrealistic, and care partners are forced to reckon with losses associated with physical limitations.

In moments like these, drawing on the experiential source of meaning is a powerful tool for you to use. For many, that bucket list includes traveling to exotic destinations. While certainly the act of getting on an airplane or train or boat itself can be exciting, more often it is not the act of travel per se that is so meaningful to us. Instead, it is the heightened connectedness to each other and the world around us through our five senses that we experience through travel that is so important. Travel allows us to connect deeply to nature, to art, and to love, each of which can be made available without the act of travel.

One of the amazing things about technology is that in many ways, we can bring the gifts of exploration right into our home. One of my patients shared that traveling to visit a favorite museum in Paris was on her mom's bucket list but getting on an airplane was unrealistic. Through some quick research she learned that several of the museums there had virtual galleries that she and her mom could visit right from their home in New Jersey. So, they spent one weekend "at the galleries," going through each painting and discussing their unique perspectives on the artist and what they saw, while eating croissants from their favorite local French bakery. They were able to connect to what was so meaningful about going to the museums in France from their living room. It wasn't travel that mattered; it was her mom's ability to connect to her love for art history, and to share that with her daughter, that mattered.

The experiential source of meaning can be your go-to tool to maximize the moments you have with your care partner now, as well as one way to cope with grief in the future. Thinking about the ways in which you and your care partner connected through experiences of the five senses, and through love, beauty, and humor can help to reinforce the connection you shared when they are no longer here. I certainly have found this to be true. I wake up each day to the classical music radio station that served as the backdrop to my relationship with my dad, keeping our tradition. On special occasions like his birthday or Father's Day, I open a bottle of Stewart's root beer, the drink we enjoyed together for decades, and imagine his smile as I take the first sip. One of my most treasured places to sit is by the shore in New Jersey where much of my childhood unfolded. I have a picture framed of the ocean from 2011, when he and I were down there staring out into the vast blue waves, on a brisk fall day. I knew when I took the picture that someday I would look at that photo and desperately long to be back in that moment. I tried to capture all elements of that moment in my mind: the sound of the ocean, the smell of the sea air, the birds flying, and most importantly, the feeling of my right hand nestled in his bony, arthritic left, my head on his shoulder, cushioned by his beige winter jacket; his breaking our hold to wipe his constantly dripping nose. Now, when I look at that picture or better yet, sit by the ocean, I can't help but think about the waves of the ocean crashing down as they had for so many moments we had together, and feel connected to him.

When I'm feeling particularly sad, I open his bottle of Aramis aftershave that I have tucked safely in the bottom of my sock drawer. Smelling it now transports me back and I'm able to connect, even just slightly so, to the joy of those moments. None of these experiences is a replacement—the pain is still sharp—but they help to soothe the still-open wound and keep our connection alive.

In Meaning-Centered Psychotherapy for Caregivers, each of these sources of meaning—*historical, attitudinal, creative, experiential*—is explored through a series of sessions in which caregivers respond to questions that bring to life how these sources of meaning can become resources, tools they can use to help them cope with the challenges of caregiving and beyond. While it can be beneficial to work with a therapist to explore the idea of meaning and caregiving, this is work that you absolutely can do on your own. At all times, the opportunity to experience meaning alongside suffering and challenge is available to us. Our job is to understand the unique and personal ways in which we can connect to meaning *despite* whatever hardships life throws our way. Working through the questions in Exercise 9.1 can help you to embrace this paradox of meaning and suffering. As you go through them, take some time to explore the ways in which each of the sources of meaning may be available to you right now.

Exercise 9.1: Questions to Facilitate Connecting to Meaning in Caregiving[19]

- As you reflect upon who you are today, what are the meaningful activities, roles, or accomplishments that you are most proud of? Is caregiving on your list? Why or why not?
- As you look toward the future, what are some of the life lessons you have learned along the way that you would want to pass on to others? How, in any way, has your caregiving journey shaped these lessons? What is the legacy you hope to live and give?
- What are some of the life limitations, losses, or obstacles you have faced in the past, and how did you cope or deal with them at the time? Since becoming a caregiver, what are the specific limitations or losses you have faced, and how are you coping or dealing with them now?

- Are you still able to find meaning in your daily life despite the limitations of caregiving and your awareness of the finiteness of life? If yes, how?
- Who are you responsible to and for? If *you* are not on that list, why might that be?
- Do you have unfinished business? What tasks have you always wanted to do but have yet to undertake? What is holding you back from doing these things?
- How do you connect with your care partner, and life more generally, through love, beauty, and humor?

✳ ✳ ✳

Robert was a sixty-four-year-old caregiver who came to see me for Meaning-Centered Psychotherapy for Caregivers. Nine months before our first session, his wife, Molly, was diagnosed with metastatic breast cancer. They had two adult daughters who lived far from where they resided. Robert previously worked full-time but reduced his hours when his wife was diagnosed, and shortly before I met him, he had taken an unpaid leave from work to attend to her growing needs. By the first session, Molly was experiencing neurocognitive changes associated with the cancer spreading to her brain, including occasional seizures, dizziness, balance and visual disturbances, speech difficulties, and incontinence. She was unable to independently complete many activities of daily living, and neither Robert nor her physicians believed it was safe for her to spend much time on her own. Robert described Molly as someone who, for their twenty-eight years of marriage, was self-sufficient and independent, took care of him, and was even-tempered. But shortly after the disease progressed to her brain, Molly had become irritable, forgetful, and even verbally aggressive. When Robert began Meaning-

Centered Psychotherapy for Caregivers, he often felt hopeless about the future, fearful of living life without his wife, and abandoned by his daughters for not being present and helping to care for their mother. Across seven sessions, we explored his identity before and after he became a caregiver, looking for ways he could utilize the sources of meaning as resources to help him cope in the present.

Historical source of meaning. As a young man, Robert had worked in his parents' restaurant and was taught from an early age an unquestionable devotion to family. The identification of this element of his past legacy helped Robert clarify why his daughters' disengagement from caring for his wife was so upsetting. He also described watching his mother take care of his father through his deterioration due to Alzheimer's disease and shared holding an old-fashioned belief in the responsibility of women to provide care, which also contributed to feelings of frustration and resentment toward his daughters. Through a discussion of current and future legacy, Robert recognized that while his past legacy had significantly impacted the value he placed on unquestionable support for family and his desire to have his daughters be more involved, he could set a new example for future generations of a more flexible attitude about traditional gender roles of care.

Attitudinal source of meaning. Robert had difficulty asking for help and accepting help when it was offered. Instead, he took on all caregiving responsibilities, in part because he believed that as a "real man" he should be able to handle things on his own. Through a discussion of how he responded to limitations and losses in the past, including his parents' deaths and a layoff from a previous job, it became clear that he had previously coped through isolating himself and hiding his emotions. He never allowed himself to cry, and when sad or scared he would remember his father saying to him as a young child to "keep a stiff upper lip," which he did. The discussion of attitude highlighted the possibility of a more vulnerable approach to caregiving. Although he was proud of how he took care of Molly, he recognized his role in making things more challenging and that he could ask his sister-in-law for help and hire a home health aide for additional support. Our discussions also highlighted the benefit of speaking openly about his feelings. Keeping a "stiff upper lip" no longer served him or his wife well, and Robert realized that although speaking about his fears openly with his wife would be painful, it would allow for increased connectedness and more shared responsibility in decision-making while it was still possible. Whereas his previous approach of concealing emotions had left him chronically worried and contributed to insomnia, the conversation about choosing his attitude underscored new ways in which he could respond to his current limitations, which would have a more positive impact on his mental and physical health.

Creative source of meaning. As a young adult, Robert had aspired to travel and cultivate his musical talents, but the need to work from a young age to contribute financially to his family prevented him from doing so. He and Molly married in their early twenties, and as soon as their first child arrived, the demands of working full-time and being an active husband and father led him to "shove those dreams away." Through an exploration of creativity, Robert identified the importance of music and his current capacity to create his life, regardless of his present challenges. He also shared his awareness that he would have life to live after his wife's death and that he could choose how to create that life. Robert realized that he did not need to wait until Molly's death to return to his dream and instead could practice the guitar and even learn to write music while spending time at home with her. Finally, this discussion highlighted ways Robert continued to create his relationship with Molly and the courage he demonstrated in opening difficult conversations with her about advance care planning. Robert felt conflicted about discussing these painful topics, but he ultimately realized that doing so would allow them both to share their feelings and feel closer to one another.

Experiential source of meaning. Since his childhood, Robert had experienced a sense of connectedness to something much greater than himself through prayer, along with a sense of awe, hope, and peace. Similarly, through music, he would often find the hours "flying by" and would get lost in the present moment. We discussed how both prayer and music could become go-to resources for him during stressful times. The discussion also highlighted the sense of peace Robert felt at night when he slept holding his wife's hand, something he had done almost every night of their marriage. Despite her limitations, in those moments Robert felt cared for, deeply loved, safe, and connected to Molly. He recognized that this connectedness was something that he could experience despite their difficult circumstances.

Through our sessions, we never denied the existence of Robert's very real challenges, the sadness of watching Molly's physical and cognitive decline, and his own anticipatory grief. However, through discussing the sources of meaning, Robert began to embrace the possibility of feeling intense pain and sadness as well as strength. He began to fully embrace the emotional crème brûlée of caregiving.

❊ ❊ ❊

You don't need to formally engage in Meaning-Centered Psychotherapy to connect to meaning and purpose in caregiving. For many, the lessons taught through the approach organically emerge. This was the case for Dr. Arthur Kleinman, who in *The Soul of Care* writes about his experience of caring for his wife with progressive Alzheimer's disease:

> It was during this time, in the last few years of caregiving, that I undertook regular exercise, slept better, created moments of genuine self-reflection, and learned to do so in the midst of many conflicting demands. After the earlier period when my health problems worsened under the stress, I worked on them (and on stress management) so conscientiously that at the close of that terrible decade, I was more robust and much healthier. I also learned how to find joy in the moment, and to relax under pressure, especially in my work life. It was a period when I deepened my ties to family and friends by actively nurturing those relationships. None of this altered the fundamental reality of Joan's constant decline and the many troubles it brought our way. The dreaded outcomes all came to pass, as we knew they would, and yet in some inexplicable way, I emerged remade.[20]

Despite recognizing the inevitable death of his wife, and despite—or perhaps better stated, in response to—an extraordinarily difficult decade of caregiving, Dr. Kleinman was able to take responsibility for his life, develop coping strategies, foster greater meaning in his relationships, and emerge more resilient, stronger, and better suited to face loss at the end of his caregiving journey than at the beginning.

I know that the relationship that I cultivated with my dad was unique. But it wasn't the nature of our relationship that ultimately drove my capacity to connect to meaning in caregiving; my ability to do so would have been just as strong had I been taking care of anyone else in my life. The challenges may have been different, as would have been the specific ways in which I experienced meaning, purpose, and growth, but the opportunity to connect to meaning would have remained. What I want to emphasize here is that you don't have to have a loving or even a healthy relationship with the person you're caring for to connect to meaning as a caregiver. What is necessary, instead, is your recognizing the possibility that meaning is available to you, despite the challenges of caregiving.

This has been the case for one of my current patients who was recently caring for her mom, with whom she had an emotionally abusive relationship as a child and adolescent. My patient, now forty-five, had spent many years in therapy working through the deep wounds caused by her mom's narcissistic tendencies. She created emotional distance and eventually became estranged from her for a decade, a period which ended when her mom reached out for help after learning of her inoperable pancreatic cancer. My patient initially was angered by this request but realized that she could either hold tightly to anger that was lingering from decades before or look at this as an opportunity to heal the relationship. She began seeing her mom weekly, but ultimately the relationship remained strained, and her mom died a few months after they reconnected. However, instead of entering grief with complicated emotions like guilt, this patient was able to reflect on how she chose her attitude in reengaging with her mom and the courage it took for her to even consider seeing her again, let alone take care of her. She was proud of herself and instead of feeling regret, she recognized through her ability to engage in caregiving, even if briefly, how much healing she had done on her own since her childhood.

Humans are complex, and this complexity is amplified by caregiving. At any one time, we may feel sadness, fear, hopelessness, anger, resentment, anxiety, and intense love for our care partner, pride in ourselves, strength, and hope. The positive and negative emotions are not mutually exclusive. Suffering and meaning can coexist. My hope is that through embracing the complexity of the human experience and the possibility for an emotional crème brûlée, you can begin—or continue—to connect to a sense of meaning and purpose as you experience the challenges of caregiving, and life.

CHAPTER 10

Stepping into the Spotlight

Stand By Me

Artist: Ben E. King
Arranged and Conducted by Stan Applebaum, 1961

String Interlude "Daphne"
Composed by Stan Applebaum, 1961

The walk home from the hospital each time after I brought my dad in became a little ritual for me. I would often leave between three and six in the morning after he had finally been admitted to a bed or at the least, had received a round of treatment in the ER and was medically stable. Regardless of the time, I'd send a text to my brother and mom, when she was still here, sharing some variation on the theme of, "It was a UTI again. He's had hydration and antibiotics and was more himself before I left." My mom would be concerned about my walking and make me promise her that I would take a cab the five blocks home, and my brother would respond, "You saved his life again."

Once in my apartment, I'd evaluate whether it was worth going to sleep given that the sun was often starting to come up, but I always attempted at least an hour of rest. I knew I would need to head back to the hospital before work, to be present when the shift change happened between 7 and 8 a.m. I'd shower and leave clothes by the door just in case I received an emergency call from the hospital in the interim and check the ringer on my phone to make sure it was up as high as possible. Then I would get into bed and take a deep inhale through my nose, and on the exhale out through my mouth I would connect to my brother's words, the words that were already deep within me. Had I not been "there," wherever "there" was, had I not been able to stand by my dad, recognizing the signs and symptoms of whatever medical process was unfolding, had I not been able to communicate clearly with him and the paramedics and the medical team, the walk home would have had a very different tone.

Had I not been present as my dad's caregiver, he would most likely have died long before 2019. And if he hadn't died, he would have experienced a quality of life that was drastically worse than the one he lived out. My presence allowed him to live his life as fully as possible for as long as possible.

Whatever form it takes for you, each time you return from a period of high-intensity caregiving, whether that is accompanying your loved one to the hospital or helping them to bathe or get dressed, I hope you will engage in a similar self-affirming ritual. Take a deep breath in, and on the exhale try to connect to the significant role you are playing and how instrumental your presence is to the quality of life of your partner in care. Doing so is one of the ultimate acts of caregiver self-care.

*   *   *

As a caregiver, you are an essential extension of the healthcare team. Today's shorter hospital stays and shift toward increased outpatient care has placed a significant burden of responsibility on you, and in most cases in the absence of formal training or support. Rapid advances in care, including new drugs and immunotherapies and more sophisticated diagnostic tools, have improved healthcare professionals' ability to extend lives and enhance survival. But this good news means that while once abruptly life-limiting illnesses are now chronic diseases, the burden on you has substantially increased.

When I began the Caregivers Clinic in 2011, one of the first caregivers I saw said to me, "What I'm doing for my mom is just as important as her chemotherapy." I completely agree. Whether you realize it or not while you're in the role, as caregivers, you have become the backbone of our healthcare system. Without a doubt, the presence of a caregiver who is dressed in invisible armor, ready to advocate on behalf of patients, negotiate our complicated healthcare system, and attempt clear and productive communication with medical, administrative, and legal professionals is not only optimal but is becoming essential to the well-being of patients today. Certainly, not all patients have caregivers. But when caregivers are available, and when they are giving all of themselves to this role, they need to be acknowledged and supported and honored. The invisibility that I often felt in the emergency room, that has been felt by so many of the caregivers with whom I have worked professionally, and that I'm certain many of you have felt, is devastating. It's detrimental to patients' well-being, caregivers' well-being, and that of our healthcare system more broadly. The more you can be formally recognized for the role that you play in the care of patients, the easier it will be for patients to receive care that is consistent with their values. The easier it will be for healthcare professionals to do their jobs. And the easier it will be for our healthcare system to function.

Standing by patients is extraordinarily difficult when done in isolation. It is nearly impossible for any one of us to shoulder all the responsibilities of taking care of a patient. As was so clear from my entire caregiving journey and those of the countless others who have shared their journeys with me, we need support on a much bigger level. We need policies that acknowledge caregiver burden as a national healthcare issue and that provide necessary infrastructure so that mental health services can be available to all caregivers in need; we need policies that recognize caregivers as key members of the healthcare team and support them in this role; we need policies that prevent caregivers from having to choose between paid employment and taking care of a loved one; and we need policies that support the home care workforce upon which we are so deeply reliant.

Until such policies are implemented, it is up to us to choose our attitude (to use a Meaning-Centered Psychotherapy term), to take control of what we can in terms of getting our needs met. Here, I outline concrete steps you can take to ensure that your needs are met, while we wait for our public policy landscape to catch up.

Training and Education in Medical and Nursing Tasks

Feeling unprepared to take responsibility for medical and nursing tasks can be a source of significant distress. Since such responsibilities often increase dramatically when patients are discharged from the hospital after a medical event or treatment, the return home from the hospital is a universally challenging one for caregivers. To address this particularly vulnerable moment, across the United States there is currently a push for caregivers to receive training *before* patients are discharged through the Caregiver Advise, Record, Enable (CARE) Act. The CARE Act standardizes hospital procedures and supports caregivers when patients transition from the hospital back to home[1] and has three provisions: It requires hospitals to record the name and contact information of caregivers in patients' medical records when they are admitted for treatment; it requires hospitals to inform caregivers when patients are to be transferred or discharged; and it requires the provision of education and training to caregivers in the medical and nursing tasks they will need to perform for patients at home. While it has not been passed at the federal level, a state-by-state approach has been taken, and to date the CARE Act has been signed into law and is either in effect or will be soon in forty-five states, the District of Columbia, Puerto Rico, and the US Virgin Islands.[2]

Regardless of whether you reside in a state where the CARE Act is active, I encourage you to speak at length with a nurse involved in your care partner's care in the hospital before they are discharged. Keep a list of all the questions you have regarding what you will have to do when you get home to take care of them. If there are certain complex medical tasks you are anxious about having to do on your own, ask the nurse to demonstrate these for you and then have them watch you do the tasks in front of them. This way you can feel confident in your ability to carry them out independently at home. Similarly, if your loved one receives home nursing care after they are discharged, take advantage of the nurses who visit and similarly have them model for you the nursing skills you're asked to perform at home, and then have them watch you do the same. Consider each visiting nurse visit an opportunity for your loved one to receive care *and* for you to receive guidance and education.

In addition to asking nurses and other staff for training, many caregivers find benefit in written materials about their loved one's illness and treatment. Since the Internet can be overwhelming with the vast amount of information out there, I suggest, instead of conducting a basic Google search, seek out medical information in one of the following ways. First, many hospitals have a Patient and Caregiver Education Department that curates illness-specific information. This is a great resource to use if it exists where your loved one receives care. Second, disease-specific organizations such as the American Cancer Society and the Alzheimer's Foundation of America have rich educational materials that have been vetted by experts. Finally, you can ask your care partner's doctor or other medical team members if they have any recommendations for reputable sources of additional information. You are more likely to be sent in a helpful direction by them than by Dr. Google.

Emotional Support

Having access to emotional support is always a good thing. However, not all of you will require or even want the level of support provided by a psychiatrist, licensed clinical psychologist, social worker, or other mental health professional. Moreover, for those of you who do require or want professional support, I know that services are not always available or affordable. For sure, the COVID-19 pandemic highlighted a mental health crisis here in the United States that was punctuated by a lack of mental health professionals with availability to take on new patients. For these reasons, my colleagues and I are passionate about building up the workforce of mental health professionals versed in supporting caregiving families so that more of you can access mental health care when you need it.

If you're lucky enough to find mental health care that's either free of charge, covered by your insurance, or otherwise affordable, since there are so many different types of support out there, it can be overwhelming to decide what type of support is best. To help you find the right type of care, here I outline some of the most common categories of services and offer some suggestions for how to connect to them.

One-on-one counseling. Speaking with a therapist one-on-one can be beneficial for a variety of reasons. Working with a therapist can give you the emotional space to share your concerns and fears and to engage in problem-solving to address caregiving-related stressors. You may find individual counseling helpful if you want to work on your ability to communicate with your care partner and members of the healthcare team. It is also the best option if you are struggling with mental health concerns, such as anxiety or depression or insomnia, that are significantly impacting your day-to-day life and your ability to carry out your caregiving responsibilities. In many cases, even just a handful of one-on-one sessions with a therapist can be helpful in improving your capacity to cope and confidence in your role. One-on-one counseling can also be invaluable if you are bereaved and struggling to manage grief in the months and years after the death of your care partner.

Family and couples counseling. Engaging in therapy as a couple or family can be incredibly powerful, especially when there are disagreements about caregiving roles or patients' and families' expectations about goals of care. For example, many caregivers who identify as the primary caregiver but who rely on support from other family members have found that engaging in a few family therapy sessions can help to clarify roles and responsibilities. If you are taking care of a spouse or partner, engaging in couples therapy can help you to navigate balancing your identity as a caregiver and your identity as a romantic partner. Additionally, opening difficult conversations about advance care planning and end-of-life care can be overwhelming to do on your own. Engaging in these conversations with the help of a therapist is one very productive approach for couples and families.

Group counseling. One of the most common concerns caregivers share with me is feeling isolated and alone; many believe that no one in their social circle understands what it's like to be a caregiver. For these reasons, support groups can be extremely beneficial. Spending time with other caregivers who understand the challenges you are facing can be validating and can help to normalize many of the feelings you might be having. Support groups are also wonderful opportunities to learn new ways of coping from others in the role.

Overall, caregivers I've worked with have had the best experiences in what are called "closed groups," that is, groups that have a set number of caregivers who join in a set number of sessions. These are differentiated from "open groups" or "drop-in" groups, where any caregiver can participate at any time. These open groups have the potential to feel overwhelming, since you may not know what to expect each week, whereas in closed groups you can get to know the other group members, develop relationships, and have set expectations about what each group meeting will be like. When looking for a support group, make sure to ask whether it will be open or closed before joining.

Medication management. While psychiatric medications are not necessary in most cases, taking an antidepressant or antianxiety medication can be extremely beneficial for some caregivers. Before beginning any psychiatric medication, it's important to first give psychotherapy a try. In fact, the therapeutic technique I discussed in detail in Chapter 3—cognitive behavioral therapy—can be just as effective or even *more* effective for some caregivers than medications in treating symptoms of anxiety and depression. However, if your symptoms are not improving after a few months of therapy, or if your symptoms are so debilitating that they are preventing you from taking care of your loved one, it can be beneficial to have your therapist refer you to a psychiatrist or psychiatric nurse practitioner who can prescribe a medication that can work alongside therapy to improve your ability to cope and your overall well-being.

Peer-to-peer support. In addition to working with a trained mental health professional individually, in a group, or via couples or family therapy, many caregivers find significant benefits in peer support. Any of you who have already been caregivers know that you are an expert on caregiving. You have a wealth of information to share and firsthand knowledge that can help other caregivers as they navigate their journeys. In fact, in many ways, this book is my way of providing that peer-to-peer support to you!

Connecting with peers, with caregiver experts, can be a wonderful way to receive additional support and information, without the challenges of finding a trained mental health professional or paying for care. There are also many online communities and apps that can connect you to other caregivers, as well as information and caregiving-specific resources. Some of these are disease specific, while others are focused on caregivers more generally. Importantly, peer support should not be considered an alternative to therapy. Instead, it is a great option as an adjunct to therapy. It may also be a great option for you if you are not experiencing any significant distress but want an understanding shoulder to lean on.

I know that finding a mental health professional to work with can be incredibly difficult, and my hope is that in the future, support programs for caregivers will be a regular offering at every medical center. I hope policies and standards will be implemented that require the development of support programs for caregivers across health systems, that provide financial support for mental health care for caregivers, and that encourage the early and repeated screening for distress so that caregivers can receive necessary care in a timely fashion. Until these policies and programs are implemented, however, it will be up to you to find support.

The first place to look for support is within the medical center where your care partner receives care. Many hospitals have staff members who provide support to caregivers, though these services are not often advertised. Therefore, it can be useful to speak with a social worker or ask a healthcare professional involved in your loved one's care about what services might be available and how best to connect with them. Second, many disease-specific community-based organizations, such as the Cancer Support Community, provide support directly to caregivers or host databases of support services available nationally. Finally, the website psychologytoday.com can be a useful tool to find a therapist in your community, especially one who takes your insurance. While as of today there is no filter on psychologytoday.com to help identify a provider who specializes in caregiver support, there is a filter for "chronic illness," and these providers likely will have the necessary expertise to support you around your caregiving-specific concerns.

Balancing Caregiving and Work

Choosing between paid employment and caregiving is a terrible decision to make, one that too many of us have faced. Almost universally, working caregivers are forced to give up sleep and time for self-care to attend to the needs of others while earning an income. Activities that would be in the service of preserving one's health are frequently neglected because there is just no available time given work and caregiving responsibilities. I've lost count of the number of caregivers who, while taking care of loved ones, were diagnosed with their own chronic or debilitating illnesses, a phenomenon mirrored by national studies of caregivers in the United States.[3] Often these diagnoses came late as caregivers struggled to make time for their own screenings and medical visits, or symptoms were misinterpreted as merely stress-related until they became so serious that medical care was urgently needed.

As of today, there are significant limitations to existing Family Medical Leave Act (FMLA) policies. The original FMLA law[4] went into effect in 1993, and in many ways, it hasn't changed much since then. To be covered under FMLA, an employee must work for an employer with fifty or more employees and have worked at their job for a minimum of one year, with at least 1,250 hours worked over the last twelve-month period. Eligible employees are entitled to twelve weeks of job-protected leave per twelve-month period to care for an immediate family member—a spouse, minor child, adult disabled child, or parent—with a serious health condition. This means that if you are the primary caregiver to a sibling or a grandparent, or to a friend or a partner to whom you are not legally married, you are currently not protected under FMLA.

FMLA can be taken as a block of time for up to twelve weeks or intermittently, in periods of whole weeks, single days, hours, and in some cases even less than an hour.[5] Intermittent FMLA may be useful if you plan to attend frequent medical appointments while maintaining your job. While FMLA is unpaid, you can use sick and vacation days to receive income during time taken via FMLA. More recently, some states have enacted laws to offer Paid Family Medical Leave (PFML), with leave time varying between four to twelve weeks. The amount of pay given varies as well, from 60 to 70 percent of workers' average weekly wages to 100 percent.

Since FMLA policies vary state by state and may shift in the future, the first step you should take when planning for time off from work either for now or in the future is to speak with an HR representative from your employer to see if job protection is available to you via FMLA. If you are in one of the few states that currently has PFML, that could make a big difference for your planning. It will be helpful to ask them whether there are any additional policies in place that might be able to assist you in the future. It's also good to get a sense of how many sick and vacation days you have stored, and whether any of these can be rolled over from year to year. Additionally, you should ask whether your employer allows colleagues to donate sick or vacation time in the case that you are running low. Some employers allow this and for several caregivers seen in the clinic, donated sick and vacation time has made a significant difference. Finally, perhaps one of the only silver linings of the COVID-19 pandemic for caregivers was that remote work became the norm, allowing caregivers whose jobs did not require in-person contact to continue to work while remaining home with care partners. If being able to work remotely would allow you to maintain both your employment and caregiving responsibilities, I encourage you to speak with your employer about having an accommodation to remain at home. Importantly, if you are under the care of a mental health professional who is supporting you in coping with the demands of caregiving, that individual can write a letter in support of such an accommodation.

Caregiver Identification and Recognition of Caregiver Status

One of the many reasons why caregivers do not receive support is that they are often not identified as caregivers or identified early enough. Until policies are implemented that systematically identify caregivers and document caregiver data, you can take a significant step in helping to shape the care you receive simply by making a point, during your annual physical exam and any other healthcare appointments, to acknowledge your caregiver status. It will be important for you to discuss the ways in which being a caregiver is impacting you medically, emotionally, and financially.

Documentation of these data will not only help you to receive the support you need but more broadly allow for the recognition that *caregiver status is a social determinant of health*. Social determinants of health are the conditions in the environments where people are born, live, learn, work, play, worship, and age that affect a wide range of health, functioning, and quality-of-life outcomes and risks. These include economic stability, education access and quality, healthcare access and quality, and social and community context. Social determinants of health have a significant impact on individuals' health and well-being, and it's time that caregiver status is recognized as one such determinant of health.

Caregiver Burden
Is a National Healthcare Issue

Throughout this book I've talked about many ways in which you can be negatively impacted by your caregiving responsibilities. In addition to anxiety, depression, and grief, a phrase that may resonate for those of you who have already been caregivers is *compassion fatigue*. Originally called secondary traumatic stress, compassion fatigue is often used to describe the experience of professionals, such as myself, of distress resulting from frequent exposure to trauma in the context of caring for others, such as repeatedly being exposed to patients who are dying or to suffering more broadly. Over time, compassion fatigue mitigates our ability to cope with the challenges of day-to-day work. Among family caregivers, compassion fatigue is not commonly labeled but very often present, especially among those in the caregiving role for more than just a few months (that is, most caregivers). Repeatedly witnessing medical emergencies in loved ones, continuously witnessing health declines in loved ones, and ultimately feeling powerless to save a loved one despite all heroic caregiving efforts made, contributes to such fatigue. Like soldiers returning from war and veterans suffering the effects years later, many of you carry a heavy emotional weight that, when left untreated, can significantly impair your capacity to resume full, healthy lives.

Burden, distress, trauma, and compassion fatigue in caregivers all represent a national healthcare crisis. The more formally this profound negative impact of caregiving on a growing number of Americans can be recognized, the greater our chances of seeing a shift in policies that seek to address caregiver training and support, mental health, and time off from work. And one way for this recognition to occur is for you to speak up. To acknowledge your caregiver status. To discuss openly with your healthcare professionals the ways in which your responsibilities are affecting all areas of your life. And to ask for help. The more vocal we can be as a community of caregivers, the greater our chance will be to be recognized for the exceptional work we do, and the support we so desperately need.

Caregivers Are Not Visitors

I was never just a visitor, and neither are you. When my dad was in the hospital, I was never there just to visit. On most occasions when we arrived at the ER, he was unable to communicate with the healthcare team without me by his side. In addition to being his surrogate communicator and decision-maker, I was also his most available aide, assisting him with eating and drinking and helping him to turn from one side of the stretcher to another to prevent bedsores. I remained on high alert for adverse events, urging staff to change diapers to prevent infections, consulting about drug side effects I had witnessed firsthand, and, once, identifying the signs of an oncoming seizure and helping him to receive timely intervention. And, undoubtedly, I provided emotional support. I was his lifeline. As you are and will be for your care partners.

It is my hope that policies will be implemented that recognize caregivers more formally as members of the healthcare team. At the very least, you should be given identification cards that allow easy entry in and out of ERs and hospitals, and notifications when the rounding team is en route to the bedside. Until such policies are enacted, it is up to you to introduce yourself to the members of the healthcare team involved in your loved one's care—typically a nurse, a medical student, a medical resident (that is, a physician still in training), and an attending physician (who leads the medical care)—and let them know that you are the patient's caregiver. Using all the communication skills and tips and tools I've provided throughout this book, share with the medical team your knowledge of your loved one's condition and let them know that you are the point person for communication. Make sure that they have your phone number and that it is documented in your care partner's medical record. These small steps early on when you get to the ER will help the team to look toward you as the person holding critical information about the patient, and someone worthy of care and respect.

✳   ✳   ✳

A fitting place to end is where I began this work in the first place, with a focus on you, the caregiver. When I began the clinic, I realized that too often, caregivers' own identities and needs were getting lost in the mix of patient care. Moreover, at that time, most research on caregivers' support needs focused on helping them to be better caregivers, not on addressing their own unique needs. My hope is that the tools I've shared will not only help you to take care of your loved one but also, importantly, help you to take care of yourself and take responsibility for your life.

Being pulled in a million directions and not having any time for yourself can leave you feeling disconnected from your sense of self. Many caregivers have told me that they don't recognize themselves, they don't recognize who they have become because of caregiving. If this is something you feel, I want you to consider what makes you authentically yourself, and whether caregiving has changed that authentic sense of self in any way. Certainly, many facets of your identity can change because of caregiving. Perhaps you are no longer able to work full- or even part-time or identify completely with your profession as you once did. Perhaps in caring for a spouse your identity as an intimate partner has been overpowered by caregiving. Perhaps you were someone who, before caregiving, was carefree, lighthearted, and energetic, and you now struggle to feel joy. Perhaps you once exercised five days a week and now feel lethargic and weakened because of your caregiving responsibilities and inability to make it to the gym regularly. Or perhaps before caregiving, you struggled with your own physical or mental health concerns, or had difficult relationships with family members, and your caregiving responsibilities made all these existing challenges exponentially more complex. In each of these scenarios, caregiving leads to very real changes—losses even. But they don't take away who you are in your core. They don't change who you are as a loving and caring person, or as someone who enjoys nature, or as someone who is a dreamer.

Remaining connected to your authentic sense of self is one of the most important things you can do to honor and preserve yourself while taking care of a loved one. For me, this meant realizing that the bars on hospital beds could dually serve as great ballet barres. Almost daily, but especially when my dad was in the hospital for more than just a few days, I would make sure to find physical and emotional space in the hospital to stretch, to point my toes, and stand tall in my body. Connecting to my forever inner ballet dancer, reviving my soul, and remembering to center and ground myself was a necessary part of those long hospital stays for me. In fact, the last picture taken of me and my dad (minus selfies taken the last evening we embraced) was of us while he was sleeping in the ICU three days before he died. I had my right leg up on the bars of his bed and was bending in his direction. I remember thinking in that moment that I would need to continue to connect to this part of myself to survive what I sensed was his impending death. And I was right. In grief, dance has served as a primary vehicle to cope with intense emotions. In fact, for the first time since 2001 when I first chose to refocus my energy from dance to healthcare, in grief I returned more seriously to my ballet practice and now spend more evenings in the studio each week than not. Dance has allowed me to reconnect with my authentic sense of self, my inner joy, my fortitude. Hours in the studio have become a new grief ritual for me now that the intensity of the initial waves has subsided. I often find myself speaking to my mom while I dance, especially when I take a class with the same teacher she studied with during the years before her death. And as I prepare to fly through the air, I imagine my dad standing by the door of the studio watching as he once did years ago.

Remaining connected to myself while I was in the thick of caregiving also meant doing my best to focus on work while I was at work, to limit the amount of sharing I did with colleagues about what was happening at home so that I could remain connected to my identity as Dr. Applebaum. Remaining connected to myself also meant being social and traveling when possible. It was an active choice to do these things. While it often meant additional pressure to find extra support for my dad when I was away and led to my anxiously checking in with the home health aides, it was well worth it, because being authentically Allison meant I couldn't watch my thirties dissipate within the walls of a hospital. Remaining connected to myself also meant dreaming of the future and setting goals, like writing this book. Remaining connected to myself meant that despite all the limitations with which I was faced, I needed to continue to live my life as fully as possible, in whatever creative way that meant.

To help you think through your authentic sense of self and the parts of your identity that have been impacted by caregiving, I encourage you to reflect on the questions in Exercise 10.1. I hope that going through these questions will highlight what became obvious to me when I first began the clinic in 2011: Despite all the ways in which our caregiving roles challenge us, inevitably we derive strength from the experience. We cultivate new skills as a result of caregiving. And who we are authentically doesn't necessarily change because of caregiving.

Exercise 10.1: Food-for-Thought Questions about Caregiving and Identity[6]

- Think about a time before you became a caregiver. From that perspective, write down four answers to the question, "Who am I?" These can be positive or negative, and include personality characteristics, beliefs, roles, things you do, etc. For example, answers might start with, "I am someone who _____" or "I am a _____."
- Now shift your perspective to the present time. How has caregiving affected your answers? How has it affected the things that are most meaningful to you?

- What are some strengths that you've gained through caregiving? What do you love most about yourself as a caregiver?
- What are the hardest parts of your caregiving role and responsibilities? When you're doing these things, do you feel proud of yourself? If not, why do you think that is?
- If a close friend was watching you perform the hardest parts of your caregiving role, what would that friend say to you?

Everyone was, is, or will be a caregiver,[7] at least once in their life, and so this is a role that touches us all. The time is now to elevate our voices as caregivers. The time is now to highlight the striking disparity between the responsibilities we are asked to assume and the support we are given in this role. The time is now to advocate for policy changes that recognize caregivers as what we truly are: invaluable members of the healthcare team.

Frequently, medical oncology colleagues of mine will share that the most productive clinical encounters occur when a caregiver is present with the patient, as that caregiver can provide a realistic picture of that patient's functioning and their health-related behaviors, from medication adherence to engagement in physical exercise and alcohol consumption. In effect, caregivers are these healthcare professionals' best friends. They have an incredibly rich and valid data set regarding the patient's functioning to share. This information on its own is beneficial, but when presented in the context of a larger story of one's life, it can have a dramatic impact on how treatment plans are developed and delivered. The downstream benefits of that caregiver's presence are vast—and extend to healthcare professionals themselves.

This, it turns out, was the case for one of my dad's physicians who I introduced in Chapter 4, who partnered in my dad's care, treated him and me and the home health aides with deep respect, and helped my dad to remain at home for the better part of his last years of life. After I shared with him the news of my dad's death, he wrote me a letter that underscored the power of our collaboration in taking care of my dad. He shared that my clear, consistent, and specific communication of my dad's goals, desires, and expectations allowed everyone who took care of him to feel like they were part of a team. The manner in which I supported my dad to communicate effectively on his own, and when that wasn't possible, the manner in which I facilitated communication, allowed this physician and many of his other healthcare team members to provide the highest level of care possible. My communication and advocacy helped them to provide this type of care. As yours will.

If I zoom out and imagine what a caregiving journey might be like ten years from now in the United States, it has the potential to be profoundly different from mine and those of many of the caregivers whose stories I have shared. If policies are implemented that establish infrastructure to support caregivers in their responsibilities, if services are developed to protect caregivers against burnout, the experience of caregiving can shift from one that often dramatically and negatively impacts all aspects of one's life to one that can be predominantly meaningful and growth-promoting. This final chapter, and this book in its entirety, is a call for caregivers to be considered a critical part of the healthcare team and supported in their role. We must stand by caregivers, as they stand by the patients who so immensely benefit from their care.

FINALE

Forever Changed by Caregiving

Sleep, Sleep, Daughter

Artist: Archie Bleyer
Music and Lyrics,
Stan Applebaum and Elsie Simmons, 1956

In the spring of 2021, a little over two years after my caregiving partnership with my dad ended, I spent a Saturday in Brooklyn with one of my closest friends at her new home. We spent the day outside in her backyard with her dog, sipping wine and marveling at a moment of calm and groundedness and hope in what had been, for both of us, a chaotic decade of caregiving and challenge. We bought three-dollar dresses at a vintage store and walked through Prospect Park. I felt normal. I felt free. We had what might be a traditional Saturday for two women in their thirties, but a day that was quite abnormal against the backdrop of what was my day-to-day life for the prior twelve years.

As the sun began to set, my friend asked if I wanted to stay and have another drink outside or head home. I can't explain what it was but there was a strong push inside me to go home. And so, I got on the train and headed back to the city. I got off on the Upper East Side and proceeded to walk toward my apartment. In front of me, maybe five or six feet, was a woman pushing an older man in a wheelchair and to her left, a frail older woman who appeared from behind to be losing her balance and about to fall. I ran over and saw that the woman pushing the wheelchair was likely around my age and was taking care of both of her aging parents. I asked if I could help her mother, and the woman seemed shocked at the offer. As if I were getting back on a bike after not riding for years, my muscle memory kicked in, and I stood in front of the older woman and steadied her with my arms, as I had done countless times with my dad. I asked her if she felt strong enough to walk, which she did, and which side she would like me to hold her up on. "Are you sure this is okay? Are you sure this isn't too much trouble?" they asked me repeatedly as we crossed slowly from one avenue to another. "Absolutely not," I said, while privately I was washed over with intense waves of emotion. Her mother and I spoke briefly during that walk. I told her it was my pleasure to walk with her, that I missed taking care of my parents, that it's a gift to have parents to take care of. She responded, "Your parents must be so proud to have you." "I lucked out in the parents department," I said back. We walked some more, taking a break here and there until the family got to their building, and then I continued to walk east toward my apartment.

What they couldn't see when I turned—or even before that with my thick N95 mask covering most of my face—was the intense emotion I was feeling. My eyes welled up with tears, and I tried to hold them in until I crossed the street but then found myself crying as I walked myself home. I felt so intensely jealous of this woman with both of her parents alive, and I wished more than anything else that the man in the wheelchair was my dad. At the same time, I felt so deeply grateful that I was there in that moment to do exactly what that woman needed, that I could help in the best way that anyone could. I entered my apartment and sobbed and realized that this was the first time since my dad's death that my caregiving identity had been triggered, that that part of myself had been activated. It was like coming home, coming back to a place of deep knowing. A place I didn't realize that I missed until that moment.

As I sat on my floor crying, I thought back to a moment, ten years earlier in 2011, when my dad was first coming down with Lewy body disease–driven autonomic changes. My mom was finishing a work dinner, and my dad was waiting outside the restaurant for her. The plan was that I would meet them after, and they would visit my new apartment that I secured along with my postdoctoral fellowship. I met my dad, and as we started to walk, he became weak and stumbled and almost fell. Thankfully, a kind man saw this happen and ran over and eventually helped us into a cab and to my apartment. I physically couldn't have gotten my dad into the cab alone, and had that man not been there, my dad would definitely have fallen and broken his hip, if not more. We would have called an ambulance, and a cycle of him being in the hospital would have been initiated.

I always had wanted to thank that man who assisted us in 2011, but I was never able to do so. As I sat on my floor in 2021, I realized that I was able to finally thank him in my own way; I was able to be for this woman what the man was for me. And I realized that that part of me, that caregiver, was still present. I also realized that while I had just had one of the most normal days of my thirties, I had been completely changed by caregiving. The prescription in my eyes was different now. What mattered was so, so very different.

* * *

During my third year of graduate school, I attended the funeral of my dad's sister. My dad and I walked into the funeral home, and I accompanied him toward the room where his sister lay in her coffin, though I didn't follow him in. When he emerged a little while later, he walked toward me, pausing to take a paper towel out of his pocket to wipe his tearful eyes and dripping nose. To his right was a small table with a bowl of hard candies, and in his typical fashion, he took a handful much larger than could ever be expected of guests. When he reached me, he put his hand in mine and with it, one of those hard candies. "It's always important to have something sweet in your mouth when you're sad," he said as we walked into the lobby.

On February 25, 2019, as I stepped onto the podium to deliver my dad's eulogy, two of my close friends passed out Werther's Original candies to all in attendance. Once I gathered the strength and courage to begin speaking, I asked everyone to open the candy and put it in their mouths. Werther's Originals were my dad's favorite, and I knew that he would want everyone to be able to taste something sweet while feeling so sad, on his account. And I wanted everyone to learn from that moment what my dad had taught me all along. What he taught me on the day of his sister's funeral; what he taught me each time he was stuck for days in the hospital and despite his limited capacity, he would make the most of his moments; what he taught me every day of his life for that matter: Life is filled with suffering and challenge, but life is also filled with meaning, with beauty, and with sweetness. He taught me to find meaning in caregiving, and in life.

I hope his legacy—this legacy—is one that you, too, will carry on.

ACKNOWLEDGMENTS

As this is a book that touches on my personal and professional caregiving journeys, there are several groups of individuals I want to thank: those who have supported the writing of this book, those who have supported my career as a caregiving scientist, and those who supported me during my caregiving journey.

The publishing process would not have begun without the generosity of *New York Times* bestselling author Jodi Kantor, who was kind enough to introduce me to my brilliant and insightful agent, Rebecca Gradinger of United Talent Agency. I am incredibly indebted to Rebecca, who masterfully coached me to take my raw, grief-driven writing and channel it into what has become this book. Rebecca stood by me during the particularly challenging time of book development during the COVID-19 lockdown and never lost faith in me or my vision for this project. I knew the moment I met my editor Leah Miller of Simon Element that she spoke the language of caregiving and truly understood how important a book like this would be. My gratitude for her editorial expertise, and that of assistant editor Emma Taussig, is unending. How fortunate I have been to have two brilliant editors to accompany me on this journey of writing. I have learned so much about writing—and myself—from Leah and Emma.

Many versions of this book were written in advance of the one you are holding. The writing and editorial process from start to finish was in all ways an exquisite road less traveled for me. I feel blessed to have traveled it, however, in extraordinary company. I am thankful for the generosity of time, energy, and honesty of Dr. Andrew Roth,

Matthew Loscalzo, Dr. Kailey Roberts, Dr. William Rosa, Alexandra Gershuny, Dr. Maria Steenkamp, Dr. Jennifer Ford, Emily Kantoff, Dr. Wendy Lichtenthal, Leah Walsh, Laura Polacek, Dr. Hannah-Rose Mitchell, Dr. Amanda Kastrinos, Morgan Loschiavo, Mia Behrens, Johannah Chase Coates, Jessica Grippo, and Carolyn Fulton. Each of these readers helped me to shape this book into one that could ultimately accomplish my goal of helping as many caregivers as possible. I am also incredibly fortunate to have had the support of Rebecca Gebert, who accompanied me masterfully throughout the entire editorial process. Like all meaningful adventures, this road included many unexpected turns, and I am grateful to Devin Goodsell for his unwavering support and for buoying me along the way.

My career in caregiving science would not have begun without my mentor, Dr. William Breitbart, who encouraged me early on to consider ways in which I could make a unique contribution to our field of psycho-oncology, who helped me to develop my career while I was overwhelmed with my caregiving responsibilities, and whose creation of Meaning-Centered Psychotherapy has inspired so much of my work. My gratitude for Bill is unending, and it is a privilege to share his Meaning-Centered Psychotherapy with the world. My career developed alongside those of two brilliant colleagues and friends, Dr. Wendy Lichtenthal, an expert in bereavement care, and Dr. Talia Zaider, an expert in family and couples therapy. I am indebted to Wendy and Talia for inspiring me to think creatively about how to address the needs of family caregivers, and for championing me through the challenges of balancing personal and professional caregiving. Together as a trio we've envisioned a world in which no family facing illness and loss remains unsupported. It's an honor to continue this work with them, which has, no doubt, only just begun.

I am deeply thankful to the many patients with whom I've had the gift of working clinically over the past fourteen years at Memorial Sloan Kettering Cancer Center. What a privilege it has been to be the recipient of these individuals' stories, vulnerability, and inner worlds, and to be trusted in their most challenging moments to hold space for suffering. My patients have taught me how resilient we are as humans, and how suffering and meaning can deeply coexist. I hope that this book, and my work more broadly, can do justice to their stories and help to create an environment in the future where many of the challenges they faced are distant memories.

As I've shared in this book, I could never have taken care of my dad and carried forward his goals of life and care without the strength, commitment, and kindness of Mark, Joel, Rolly, Eric, and every other home health aide who formed an absolute dream team of care for my dad. Without them, I would not have been able to continue working and would never have accomplished as much as I have professionally while taking care of my dad. These extraordinary humans became my dad's family, as well as mine. Each is a superhero without a cape, and each deserves to be honored as such.

Undoubtedly, there are a few other superheroes who need mentioning. When I think about my last decade of caregiving and loss, I reflect on how blessed I've been to have had the most incredible tribe surrounding and supporting me. Jess always reminded me to keep dancing in the rain. Alex helped me to find laughter in the darkness. Trista encouraged me to explore the depths of my soul. Maria made certain I never felt alone. And Johannah ensured that I never lost sight of who I was, and who I wanted to be in this world. Finally, I look back with profound gratitude for Kamran, who stood firmly by me as I stood by my dad.

FURTHER READING

The following books are phenomenal resources to help you on your journey of coping with the challenges of caregiving:

Brach, Tara. *Radical Acceptance: Embracing Your Life with the Heart of a Buddha.* New York: Penguin Random House, 2004.

Brach, Tara. *Radical Compassion: Learning to Love Yourself and Your World with the Practice of RAIN.* New York: Penguin Life, 2020.

Cacciatore, Joanne. *Bearing the Unbearable: Love, Loss, and the Heartbreaking Path of Grief.* Somerville, MA: Wisdom Publications, 2017.

Chodron, Pema. *Comfortable with Uncertainty: 108 Teachings on Cultivating Fearlessness and Compassion.* Boulder, CO: Shambhala, 2003.

Chodron, Pema. *Welcoming the Unwelcome: Wholehearted Living in a Brokenhearted World.* Boulder, CO: Shambhala, 2020.

Chodron, Pema. *When Things Fall Apart: Heart Advice for Difficult Times.* Boulder, CO: Shambhala, 2016.

Frankl, Viktor E. *Man's Search for Meaning*. Boston: Beacon Press, 2006.

Lakshmin, Pooja. *Real Self-Care: A Transformative Program for Redefining Wellness (Crystals, Cleanses, and Bubble Baths Not Included)*. New York: Penguin Life, 2023.

Mannix, Kathryn. *Listen: How to Find the Words for Tender Conversations*. Glasgow: William Collins, 2022.

Mannix, Kathryn. *With the End in Mind: Dying, Death, and Wisdom in an Age of Denial*. Boston: Little, Brown Spark, 2018.

May, Katherine. *Wintering: The Power of Rest and Retreat in Difficult Times*. New York: Riverhead Books, 2020.

If you are interested in reading more about caregiving and our healthcare system, I highly recommend the following:

Chen, Pauline W. *Final Exam: A Surgeon's Reflections on Mortality*. New York: Vintage, 2008.

Cohan, Deborah J. *Welcome to Wherever We Are: A Memoir of Family, Caregiving, and Redemption*. New Brunswick, NJ: Rutgers University Press, 2020.

Epstein, Ronald. *Attending: Medicine, Mindfulness, and Humanity*. New York: Scribner, 2017.

Fins, Joseph J. *Rights Come to Mind: Brain Injury, Ethics, and the Struggle for Consciousness.* Cambridge: Cambridge University Press, 2015.

Gawande, Atul. *Being Mortal: Medicine and What Matters in the End.* New York: Metropolitan Books, 2014.

Kalanithi, Paul. *When Breath Becomes Air.* New York: Penguin Random House, 2016.

Karlawish, Jason. *The Problem of Alzheimer's: How Science, Culture, and Politics Turned a Rare Disease into a Crisis and What We Can Do About It.* New York: St. Martin's Griffin, 2022.

Kleinman, Arthur. *The Soul of Care: The Moral Education of a Husband and a Doctor.* London: Penguin Books Ltd, 2020.

Loscalzo, Matthew, Linda Klein, and Marshall Forstein. *Loss and Grief: Personal Stories of Doctors and Other Healthcare Professionals.* New York: Oxford University Press, 2022.

Poo, Ai-jen. *The Age of Dignity: Preparing for the Elder Boom in a Changing America.* New York: The New Press, 2016.

NOTES

Prelude:
The Causality Dilemma of Caregiving

Allison's Theme

1. Melissa Matson, Lixin Song, and Deborah K. Mayer, "Putting To-gether the Pieces of the Puzzle: Identifying Existing Evidence-Based Resources to Support the Cancer Caregiver," *Clinical Journal of Oncology Nursing* 18, no. 6 (December 2014): 619–21, https://doi.org/10.1188/14.Cjon.619-621.

Chapter 1:
Becoming a Storyteller

Passing Strangers

1. Francis W. Peabody, "The Care of the Patient," *Journal of the American Medical Association* 252, no. 6 (August 10, 1984): 813–18, https://doi.org/10.1001/jama.252.6.813.
2. Atul Gawande, *Being Mortal: Medicine and What Matters in the End* (New York: Metropolitan Books, 2014), 141.
3. Arthur Kleinman, *The Soul of Care: The Moral Education of a Hus-band and a Doctor* (London: Penguin Books Ltd, 2020), 210.

Chapter 2:
Embracing the Change

Goodbye Summer

1. AARP and National Alliance for Caregiving, *Caregiving in the United States 2020* (Washington, DC: AARP, May 2020), https://doi.org/10.26419/ppi.00103.001.
2. Ibid.
3. Ibid.
4. Ibid.
5. María P. Aranda and Bob G. Knight, "The Influence of Ethnicity and Culture on the Caregiver Stress and Coping Process: A Sociocultural Review and Analysis," *Gerontologist* 37, no. 3 (June 1997): 342–54, https://doi.org/10.1093/geront/37.3.342; M. Powell Lawton, Doris Rajagopal, Elaine Brody, and Morton H. Kleban, "The Dynamics of Caregiving for a Demented Elder among Black and White Families," *Journal of Gerontology* 47, no. 4 (July 1992): 156–64, https://doi.org/10.1093/geronj/47.4.S156; Bob G. Knight, Gia S. Robinson, Crystal V. Flynn Longmire, Miae Chun, Kayoko Nakao, and Jung Hyun Kim, "Cross Cultural Issues in Caregiving for Persons with Dementia: Do Familism Values Reduce Burden and Distress?" *Ageing International* 27, no. 3 (June 2002): 70–94, https://doi.org/10.1007/s12126-003-1003-y; and Bob G. Knight and Philip Sayegh, "Cultural Values and Caregiving: The Updated Sociocultural Stress and Coping Model," *The Journals of Gerontology: Series B* 65, no. 1 (January 2010): 5–13, https://doi.org/10.1093/geronb/gbp096.
6. National Center on Caregiving, *Women and Caregiving: Facts and Figures* (San Francisco: Family Caregiver Alliance, 2003),

https://www.caregiver.org/resource/women-and-caregiving
-facts-and-figures/; Martin Pinquart and Silvia Sörensen, "Gender Differences in Caregiver Stressors, Social Resources, and
Health: An Updated Meta-Analysis," *The Journals of Gerontology:
Series B* 61, no. 1 (January 2006): 33–45, https://doi.org/10.1093
/geronb/61.1.p33; Nidhi Sharma, Subho Chakrabarti, and San-
deep Grover, "Gender Differences in Caregiving among Family-
Caregivers of People with Mental Illnesses," *World Journal of
Psychiatry* 6, no. 1 (March 2016): 7–17, https://dx.doi.org/10.5498
/wjp.v6.i1.7; and Madson A. Maximiano-Barreto, Ludmyla C.
de Souza Alves, Diana Q. Monteiro, Aline C. M. Gratão, Sofia
C. I. Pavarini, Bruna M. Luchesi, and Marcos H. N. Chagas, "Cultural Factors Associated with Burden in Unpaid Caregivers of
Older Adults: A Systematic Review," *Health and Social Care in
the Community* (September 2022): 1–14, https://doi.org/10.1111
/hsc.14003.

7. AARP and National Alliance for Caregiving, *Caregiving in the
United States 2020.*

8. Kristin Litzelman, "The Unique Experience of Caregivers Based
on Their Life Stage and Relationship to the Patient," in Allison J.
Applebaum, ed., *Cancer Caregivers* (New York: Oxford University
Press, 2019), 34–49.

9. Nadine F. Marks, "Caregiving across the Lifespan: National Prevalence and Predictors," *Family Relations: An Interdisciplinary Journal of Applied Family Studies* 45 (January 1996): 27–36, https://
doi.org/10.2307/584767.

10. Mary Dellmann-Jenkins, Maureen Blankemeyer, and Odessa
Pinkard, "Young Adult Children and Grandchildren in Primary
Caregiver Roles to Older Relatives and Their Service Needs,"
*Family Relations: An Interdisciplinary Journal of Applied Fam-
ily Studies* 49 (February 2004): 177–86, https://doi.org/10.1111

/j.1741-3729.2000.00177.x; and Mary Dellmann-Jenkins, Maureen Blankemeyer, and Odessa Pinkard, "Incorporating the Elder Caregiving Role into the Developmental Tasks of Young Adulthood," *The International Journal of Aging and Human Development* 52, no. 1 (January 2001): 1–18, https://doi.org/10.2190/fgqa-65fu-jgnt-6c9j.

11. Women's Institute for a Secure Retirement, *Caregivers: Care for Yourself While Caring for Others* (Washington, DC: WISER, 2009), https://www.alz.org/media/sewi/documents/wiser_caregivers-_care_for_yourself_while_caring_for_others.pdf; Women's Institute for a Secure Retirement, *The Effects of Caregiving* (Washington, DC: WISER, 2012), https://wiserwomen.org/wp-content/uploads/2019/11/effects-of-caregiving-2012.pdf; and Norah Keating, Janet Fast, Donna Lero, Sarah Lucas, and Jacquie Eales, "A Taxonomy of the Economic Costs of Family Care to Adults," *The Journal of the Economics of Ageing* 3 (April 2014): 11–20, https://doi.org/10.1016/j.jeoa.2014.03.002.

12. Litzelman, "The Unique Experience of Caregivers Based on Their Life Stage and Relationship to the Patient."

13. Dellmann-Jenkins, Blankemeyer, and Pinkard, "Young Adult Children and Grandchildren in Primary Caregiver Roles to Older Relatives and Their Service Needs."

14. Dellmann-Jenkins, Blankemeyer, and Pinkard, "Incorporating the Elder Caregiving Role into the Developmental Tasks of Young Adulthood."

15. Dellmann-Jenkins, Blankemeyer, and Pinkard, "Young Adult Children and Grandchildren in Primary Caregiver Roles to Older Relatives and Their Service Needs."

16. Dellmann-Jenkins, Blankemeyer, and Pinkard, "Incorporating the Elder Caregiving Role into the Developmental Tasks of Young Adulthood."

17. Jenny Puterman and Susan Cadell, "Timing Is Everything: The Experience of Parental Cancer for Young Adult Daughters—A Pilot Study," *Journal of Psychosocial Oncology* 26 (October 2008): 103–21, https://doi.org/10.1300/J077v26n02_07.

18. Litzelman, "The Unique Experience of Caregivers Based on Their Life Stage and Relationship to the Patient."

19. Lydia Saad, "Chronic Illness Rates Swell in Middle Age, Taper Off after 75," *Gallup*, April 29, 2011, https://news.gallup.com/poll/147317/chronic-illness-rates-swell-middle-age-taper-off.aspx.

20. Julie C. Lima, Susan M. Allen, Frances Goldscheider, and Orna Intrator, "Spousal Caregiving in Late Midlife Versus Older Ages: Implications of Work and Family Obligations," *The Journals of Gerontology: Series B* 63, no. 4 (July 2008): 229–38, https://doi.org/10.1093/geronb/63.4.S229.

21. Janet Harden, "Developmental Life Stage and Couples' Experiences with Prostate Cancer: A Review of the Literature," *Cancer Nursing* 28, no. 2 (March 2005): 85–98, https://doi.org/10.1097/00002820-200503000-00002.

22. Barbara Given and Charles Given, "The Burden of Caregivers," in Allison J. Applebaum, ed., *Cancer Caregivers* (New York: Oxford University Press, 2019), 20–33.

23. Ibid.; Youngmee Kim, Kelly M. Shaffer, Charles S. Carver, and Rachel S. Cannady, "Prevalence and Predictors of Depressive Symptoms among Cancer Caregivers 5 Years after the Relative's Cancer Diagnosis," *Journal of Consulting and Clinical Psychology* 82, no. 1 (February 2014): 1–8, https://doi.org/10.1037/a0035116; Hai-Mei Geng, Dong-Mei Chuang, Fang Yang, Yang Yang, Wei-Min Liu, Li-Hui Liu, and Hong-Mei Tian, "Prevalence and Determinants of Depression in Caregivers of Cancer Patients: A Systematic Review and Meta-Analysis," *Medicine*

97, no. 39 (September 2018): e11863, https://doi.org/10.1097
/md.0000000000011863; and Rafael Del-Pino-Casado, Emilia
Priego-Cubero, Catalina López-Martínez, and Vasiliki Orgeta,
"Subjective Caregiver Burden and Anxiety in Informal Caregiv-
ers: A Systematic Review and Meta-Analysis," *PLoS One* 16, no. 3
(March 2021), https://doi.org/10.1371/journal.pone.0247143.

24. Kelly M. Shaffer, Youngmee Kim, and Charles S. Carver, "Physical and Mental Health Trajectories of Cancer Patients and Caregivers across the Year Post-Diagnosis: A Dyadic Investigation,"
Psychology and Health 31, no. 6 (June 2016): 655–74, https://doi
.org/10.1080/08870446.2015.1131826; Kelly M. Shaffer, Youngmee Kim, Charles S. Carver, and Rachel S. Cannady, "Effects of
Caregiving Status and Changes in Depressive Symptoms on
Development of Physical Morbidity among Long-Term Cancer
Caregivers," *Health Psychology* 36, no. 8 (August 2017): 770–78,
https://doi.org/10.1037/hea0000528; and Kelly M. Shaffer,
Youngmee Kim, Charles S. Carver, and Rachel S. Cannady, "De-
pressive Symptoms Predict Cancer Caregivers' Physical Health
Decline," *Cancer* 123, no. 21 (November 2017): 4277–85, https://
doi.org/10.1002/cncr.30835.

25. Ji Jianguang, Bengt Zöller, Kristina Sundquist, and Jan Sundquist, "Increased Risks of Coronary Heart Disease and Stroke
among Spousal Caregivers of Cancer Patients," *Circulation* 125,
no. 14 (April 2012): 1742–47, https://doi.org/10.1161/circulation
aha.111.057018.

26. Youngmee Kim, Charles S. Carver, Kelly M. Shaffer, Ted Gansler,
and Rachel S. Cannady, "Cancer Caregiving Predicts Physical
Impairments: Roles of Earlier Caregiving Stress and Being a
Spousal Caregiver," *Cancer* 121, no. 2 (January 2015): 302–10,
https://doi.org/10.1002/cncr.29040.

27. Kirstin F. Maltby, Christine R. Sanderson, Elizabeth A. Lobb,

and Jane L. Phillips, "Sleep Disturbances in Caregivers of Patients with Advanced Cancer: A Systematic Review," *Palliative and Supportive Care* 15, no. 1 (February 2017): 125–40, https://doi.org/10.1017/s1478951516001024; and Glenna S. Brewster, Dingyue Wang, Miranda V. McPhillips, Fayron Epps, and Irene Yang, "Correlates of Sleep Disturbance Experienced by Informal Caregivers of Persons Living with Dementia: A Systematic Review," *Clinical Gerontologist* (October 2022): 1–28, https://doi.org/10.1080/07317115.2022.2139655.

28. James M. Trauer, Mary Y. Qian, Joseph S. Doyle, Shantha M. Rajaratnam, and David Cunnington, "Cognitive Behavioral Therapy for Chronic Insomnia: A Systematic Review and Meta-Analysis," *Annals of Internal Medicine* 163, no. 3 (August 2015): 191–204, https://doi.org/10.7326/m14-2841.

29. Bruce Horovitz, "New AARP Report Finds Family Caregivers Provide $600 Billion in Unpaid Care Across the U.S.," AARP, March 8, 2023, https://www.aarp.org/caregiving/financial-legal/info-2023/unpaid-caregivers-provide-billions-in-care.html.

30. Martin L. Brown and Robin Yabroff, "Economic Impact of Cancer in the United States," in David Schottenfeld and Joseph F. Fraumeni, eds., *Cancer Epidemiology and Prevention* (New York: Oxford University Press, 2006).

31. Beverley M. Essue, Nicolas Iragorri, Natalie Fitzgerald, and Claire de Oliveira, "The Psychosocial Cost Burden of Cancer: A Systematic Literature Review," *Psycho-Oncology* 29, no. 11 (November 2020): 1746–60, https://doi.org/10.1002/pon.5516.

32. Nicolas Iragorri, Claire de Oliveira, Natalie Fitzgerald, and Beverley Essue, "The Out-of-Pocket Cost Burden of Cancer Care—A Systematic Literature Review," *Current Oncology* 28, no. 2 (March 2021): 1216–48, https://www.mdpi.com/1718-7729/28/2/117.

33. Benjamin B. Albright, Roni Nitecki, Fumiko Chino, Junzo P. Chino, Laura J. Havrilesky, Emeline M. Aviki, and Haley A. Moss, "Catastrophic Health Expenditures, Insurance Churn, and Nonemployment among Gynecologic Cancer Patients in the United States," *American Journal of Obstetrics and Gynecology* 226, no. 3 (March 2022): 384.e1–e13, https://doi.org/10.1016/j .ajog.2021.09.034.

34. John W. Scott, Nakul P. Raykar, John A. Rose, Thomas C. Tsai, Cheryl K. Zogg, Adil H. Haider, Ali Salim, John G. Meara, and Mark G. Shrime, "Cured into Destitution: Catastrophic Health Expenditure Risk among Uninsured Trauma Patients in the United States," *Annals of Surgery* 267, no. 6 (June 2018): 1093–99, https://doi.org/10.1097/sla.0000000000002254.

35. Ke Xu, David B. Evans, Kei Kawabata, Riadh Zeramdini, Jan Klavus, and Christopher J. Murray, "Household Catastrophic Health Expenditure: A Multicountry Analysis," *Lancet* 362, no. 9378 (July 2003): 111–17, https://doi.org/10.1016/s0140-6736(03)13861-5.

36. AARP and National Alliance for Caregiving, *Caregiving in the United States 2020.*

37. Chizuko Wakabayashi and Katharine M. Donato, "Does Caregiving Increase Poverty among Women in Later Life? Evidence from the Health and Retirement Survey," *Journal of Health and Social Behavior* 47, no. 3 (September 2006): 258–74, https://doi.org /10.1177/002214650604700305.

38. Metlife Mature Market Institute, *The Metlife Study of Caregiving Costs to Working Caregivers: Double Jeopardy for Baby Boomers Caring for Their Parents* (Westport, CT: Metlife, 2011), https:// www.caregiving.org/wp-content/uploads/2011/06/mmi-caregiv ing-costs-working-caregivers.pdf.

39. AARP and National Alliance for Caregiving, *Caregiving in the United States 2020.*

40. Ibid.

41. Laurie Chassin, Jon T. Macy, Dong-Chul Seo, Clark C. Presson, and Steven J. Sherman, "The Association between Membership in the Sandwich Generation and Health Behaviors: A Longitudinal Study," *Journal of Applied Developmental Psychology* 31, no. 1 (January 2010): 38–46, https://doi.org/10.1016/j.appdev.2009.06.001.

42. Elizabeth A. Perkins and William E. Haley, "Compound Caregiving: When Lifelong Caregivers Undertake Additional Caregiving Roles," *Rehabilitation Psychology* 55 (November 2010): 409–17, https://doi.org/10.1037/a0021521.

43. Youngmee Kim and Richard Schulz, "Family Caregivers' Strains: Comparative Analysis of Cancer Caregiving with Dementia, Diabetes, and Frail Elderly Caregiving," *Journal of Aging and Health* 20, no. 5 (August 2008): 483–503, https://doi.org/10.1177/0898264308317533.

44. Erin E. Kent, Katherine A. Ornstein, and J. Nicholas Dionne-Odom, "The Family Caregiving Crisis Meets an Actual Pandemic," *Journal of Pain and Symptom Management* 60, no. 1 (July 2020): e66–e69, https://doi.org/10.1016/j.jpainsymman.2020.04.006.

45. Seema Mishra, Abhity Gulia, and Sushma Bhatnagar, "Multiple Caregiving Role with the Novel Challenge of Covid-19 Pandemic: A Crisis Situation," *Indian Journal of Palliative Care* 26, Supplement 1 (June 2020): 163–65, https://doi.org/10.4103/ijpc.Ijpc_165_20; and Prajakta Dhavale, Akhila Koparkar, and Prakash Fernandes, "Palliative Care Interventions from a Social Work Perspective and the Challenges Faced by Patients and Caregivers During Covid-19," *Indian Journal of Palliative Care* 26, Supplement 1 (June 2020): 58–62, https://doi.org/10.4103/ijpc.Ijpc_149_20.

46. Supriya Mohile et al., "Perspectives from the Cancer and Aging Research Group: Caring for the Vulnerable Older Patient with

Cancer and Their Caregivers During the Covid-19 Crisis in the United States," *Journal of Geriatric Oncology* 11, no. 5 (June 2020): 753–60, https://doi.org/10.1016/j.jgo.2020.04.010.

47. AARP and National Alliance for Caregiving, *Caregiving in the United States 2020*.

Chapter 3:
A Master Class in Mindfulness

This Magic Moment

1. Atul Gawande, *Being Mortal: Medicine and What Matters in the End* (New York: Metropolitan Books, Henry Holt and Company, 2014).

2. "Mr. Men, Little Miss," THOIP, accessed February 14, 2022, https://mrmen.com/.

3. NIMH Information Resource Center, "Generalized Anxiety Disorder," accessed December 7, 2022, https://www.nimh.nih.gov/health/statistics/generalized-anxiety-disorder.

4. Adapted from Michael H. Antoni, *Stress Management Intervention for Women with Breast Cancer: Participant's Workbook* (Washington, DC: American Psychological Association, 2003).

5. Aaron T. Beck, "The Current State of Cognitive Therapy: A 40-Year Retrospective," *Archives of General Psychiatry* 62, no. 9 (September 2005): 953–59, https://doi.org/10.1001/archpsyc.62.9.953; and Aaron T. Beck, "A 60-Year Evolution of Cognitive Theory and Therapy," *Perspectives on Psychological Science* 14, no. 1 (January 2019): 16–20, https://doi.org/10.1177/1745691618804187.

6. Stefan G. Hofmann and Jasper A. J. Smits, "Cognitive-Behavioral Therapy for Adult Anxiety Disorders: A Meta-

Analysis of Randomized Placebo-Controlled Trials," *Journal of Clinical Psychiatry* 69, no. 4 (April 2008): 621–32, https://doi.org/10.4088/jcp.v69n0415; Pim Cuijpers, Matthias Berking, Gerhard Andersson, Leanne Quigley, Annet Kleiboer, and Keith S. Dobson, "A Meta-Analysis of Cognitive-Behavioural Therapy for Adult Depression, Alone and in Comparison with Other Treatments," *Canadian Journal of Psychiatry* 58, no. 7 (July 2013): 376–85, https://doi.org/10.1177/070674371305800702; Stefan G. Hofmann, Joshua Curtiss, Joseph K. Carpenter, and Shelley Kind, "Effect of Treatments for Depression on Quality of Life: A Meta-Analysis," *Cognitive Behaviour Therapy* 46, no. 4 (June 2017): 265–86, https://doi.org/10.1080/16506073.2017.1304445; and Joseph K. Carpenter, Leigh A. Andrews, Sara M. Witcraft, Mark B. Powers, Jasper A. J. Smits, and Stefan G. Hofmann, "Cognitive Behavioral Therapy for Anxiety and Related Disorders: A Meta-Analysis of Randomized Placebo-Controlled Trials," *Depression and Anxiety* 35, no. 6 (June 2018): 502–14, https://doi.org/10.1002/da.22728.

7. Joseph Wolpe, *The Practice of Behavior Therapy* (New York: Pergamon, 1973).

8. Tomer T. Levin and Allison J. Applebaum, "Acute Cancer Cognitive Therapy," *Cognitive and Behavioral Practice* 21 (November 2014): 404–15, https://doi.org/10.1016/j.cbpra.2014.03.003; and Jamie Jacobs, Lara Traeger, Emily Walsh, and Joseph Greer, "Cognitive Behavioral Therapy for Informal Cancer Caregivers," in Allison J. Applebaum, ed., *Cancer Caregivers* (New York: Oxford University Press, 2019), 149–63.

9. Levin and Applebaum, "Acute Cancer Cognitive Therapy."

10. Adapted from Joseph Greer, Jessica Graham, and Steven Safren, "Resolving Treatment Complications Associated with Comorbid Medical Conditions," in Michael Otto and Stefan Hofmann,

eds., *Avoiding Treatment Failures in the Anxiety Disorders* (New York: Springer, 2010), 317–46.

11. Ai-jen Poo and Ariane Conrad, *The Age of Dignity: Preparing for the Elder Boom in a Changing America* (New York: The New Press, 2015), 124.

12. Tara Brach, "Tara Brach," accessed December 7, 2022, https://www.tarabrach.com/.

13. Adapted from David H. Barlow and Michelle G. Craske, *Mastery of Your Anxiety and Panic: Workbook*, 5th edition (New York: Oxford University Press, 2022).

Chapter 4: Combating Ageism and Other Forms of Discrimination

I Can Tell The Way You Say Hello

1. Diverse Elders Coalition, *Caring for Those Who Care. Resources for Providers: Meeting the Needs of Diverse Family Caregivers* (Washington, DC: Diverse Elders Coalition, 2021), https://www.diverseelders.org/wp-content/uploads/2021/03/DEC-Toolkit-Final-R2.pdf.

2. World Health Organization, *Global Report on Ageism* (Geneva, Switzerland: World Health Organization, 2021), https://www.who.int/publications/i/item/9789240016866.

3. Tina Reed, "Boomers' Caregiving Crisis," *Axios*, November 19, 2022, https://www.axios.com/2022/11/19/baby-boomers-elder-care.

4. James R. Knickman and Emily K. Snell, "The 2030 Problem: Caring for Aging Baby Boomers," *Health Services Research* 37, no. 4 (August 2002): 849–84, https://doi.org/10.1034/j.1600-0560.2002.56.x.

5. AARP and National Alliance for Caregiving, *Caregiving in the United States 2020* (Washington, DC: AARP, 2020), https://doi.org/10.26419/ppi.00103.001.

6. Bernice Neugarten, *Middle Age and Aging* (Chicago: The University of Chicago Press, 1968); and Theris Touhy and Kathleen F. Jett, *Ebersole and Hess's Toward Healthy Aging: Human Needs and Nursing Responses* (Maryland Heights, MO: Elsevier, 2012).

7. José Manuel Sousa São José, Carla Alexandra Filipe Amado, Stefania Ilinca, Sandra Catherine Buttigieg, and Annika Taghizadeh Larsson, "Ageism in Health Care: A Systematic Review of Operational Definitions and Inductive Conceptualizations," *Gerontologist* 59, no. 2 (March 2019): 98–108, https://doi.org/10.1093/geront/gnx020.

8. Liat Ayalon and Amber M. Gum, "The Relationships between Major Lifetime Discrimination, Everyday Discrimination, and Mental Health in Three Racial and Ethnic Groups of Older Adults," *Aging and Mental Health* 15, no. 5 (July 2011): 587–94, https://doi.org/10.1080/13607863.2010.543664; and Lisa L. Barnes, Carlos F. Mendes de Leon, Robert S. Wilson, Julia L. Bienias, David A. Bennett, and Denis A. Evans, "Racial Differences in Perceived Discrimination in a Community Population of Older Blacks and Whites," *Journal of Aging and Health* 16, no. 3 (June 2004): 315–37, https://doi.org/10.1177/0898264304264202.

9. Tené T. Lewis, Lisa L. Barnes, Julia L. Bienias, Daniel T. Lackland, Denis A. Evans, and Carlos F. Mendes de Leon, "Perceived Discrimination and Blood Pressure in Older African American and White Adults," *Journals of Gerontology Series A* 64, no. 9 (September 2009): 1002–8, https://doi.org/10.1093/gerona/glp062; Briana Mezuk, Kiarri N. Kershaw, Darrell Hudson, Kyuang Ah Lim, and Scott Ratliff, "Job Strain, Workplace Discrimination, and Hypertension among Older Workers: The Health and Retirement Study,"

Race and Social Problems 3, no. 1 (March 2011): 38–50, https://doi .org/10.1007/s12552-011-9041-7; and Ye Luo, Jun Xu, Ellen Granberg, and William M. Wentworth, "A Longitudinal Study of Social Status, Perceived Discrimination, and Physical and Emotional Health among Older Adults," *Research on Aging* 34, no. 3 (May 2011): 275–301, https://doi.org/10.1177/0164027511 426151.

10. Leslie R. M. Hausmann, Michael J. Hannon, Denise M. Kresevic, Barbara H. Hanusa, C. Kent Kwoh, and Said A. Ibrahim, "Impact of Perceived Discrimination in Healthcare on Patient-Provider Communication," *Medical Care* 49, no. 7 (July 2011): 626–33, https://doi.org/10.1097/MLR.0b013e318215d93c.

11. Amal N. Trivedi and John Z. Ayanian, "Perceived Discrimination and Use of Preventive Health Services," *Journal of General Internal Medicine* 21, no. 6 (June 2006): 553–58, https://doi .org/10.1111/j.1525-1497.2006.00413.x.

12. Amy B. Dailey, Stanislav V. Kasl, Theodore R. Holford, and Beth A. Jones, "Perceived Racial Discrimination and Nonadherence to Screening Mammography Guidelines: Results from the Race Differences in the Screening Mammography Process Study," *American Journal of Epidemiology* 165, no. 11 (June 2007): 1287–95, https://doi.org/10.1093/aje/kwm004; Leslie R. M. Hausmann, Kwonho Jeong, James E. Bost, and Said A. Ibrahim, "Perceived Discrimination in Health Care and Use of Preventive Health Services," *Journal of General Internal Medicine* 23, no. 10 (October 2008): 1679–84, https://doi.org/10.1007/s11606-008-0730-x; and LaVera M. Crawley, David K. Ahn, and Marilyn A. Winkleby, "Perceived Medical Discrimination and Cancer Screening Behaviors of Racial and Ethnic Minority Adults," *Cancer Epidemiology, Biomarkers and Prevention*, no. 8 (August 2008): 1937–44, https://doi.org/10.1158/1055-9965.epi-08-0005.

13. Courtney Van Houtven, Corrine I. Voils, Eugene Z. Oddone, Kevin P. Weinfurt, Joëlle Y. Friedman, Kevin A. Schulman, and Hayden B. Bosworth, "Perceived Discrimination and Reported Delay of Pharmacy Prescriptions and Medical Tests," *Journal of General Internal Medicine* 20, no. 7 (July 2005): 578–83, https://www.ncbi.nlm.nih.gov/pmc/articles/PMC1490147/.

14. Steven M. Asch, Elizabeth M. Sloss, Christopher Hogan, Robert H. Brook, and Richard L. Kravitz, "Measuring Underuse of Necessary Care among Elderly Medicare Beneficiaries Using Inpatient and Outpatient Claims," *Journal of the American Medical Association* 284, no. 18 (November 2000): 2325–33, https://doi.org/10.1001/jama.284.18.2325; Jibby E. Kurichi, Liliana Pezzin, Joel E. Streim, Pui L. Kwong, Ling Na, Hillary R. Bogner, Dawei Xie, and Sean Hennessy, "Perceived Barriers to Healthcare and Receipt of Recommended Medical Care among Elderly Medicare Beneficiaries," *Archives of Gerontology and Geriatrics* 72 (September 2017): 45–51, https://doi.org/10.1016/j.archger.2017.05.007; and Centers for Disease Control and Prevention, Administration on Aging, Agency for Healthcare Research and Quality, and Centers for Medicare and Medicaid Services, *Enhancing Use of Clinical Preventive Services Among Older Adults* (Washington, DC: AARP, 2011), https://www.cdc.gov/aging/pdf/Clinical_Preventive_Services_Closing_the_Gap_Report.pdf.

15. Katherine Corcoran, Justin McNab, Seham Girgis, and Ruth Colagiuri, "Is Transport a Barrier to Healthcare for Older People with Chronic Diseases?" *Asia Pacific Journal of Health Management* 7 (January 2012): 49–56, https://www.researchgate.net/publication/306225275_Is_Transport_a_Barrier_to_Healthcare_for_Older_People_with_Chronic_Diseases; and R. Turner Goins, Kimberly A. Williams, Mary W. Carter, Melinda Spencer,

and Tatiana Solovieva, "Perceived Barriers to Health Care Access among Rural Older Adults: A Qualitative Study," *Journal of Rural Health* 21, no. 3 (June 2006): 206–13, https://doi .org/10.1111/j.1748-0361.2005.tb00084.x.

16. Ayalon and Gum, "The Relationships between Major Lifetime Discrimination, Everyday Discrimination, and Mental Health in Three Racial and Ethnic Groups of Older Adults"; Barnes, Mendes de Leon, Wilson, Bienias, Bennett, and Evans, "Racial Differences in Perceived Discrimination in a Community Population of Older Blacks and Whites"; Lewis, Barnes, Bienias, Lackland, Evans, and Mendes de Leon, "Perceived Discrimination and Blood Pressure in Older African American and White Adults"; and Mezuk, Kershaw, Hudson, Lim, and Ratliff, "Job Strain, Workplace Discrimination, and Hypertension among Older Workers."

17. Timothy W. Farrell et al., "Exploring the Intersection of Structural Racism and Ageism in Healthcare," *Journal of the American Geriatrics Society* 70, no. 12 (December 2022): 3366–77, https:// doi.org/10.1111/jgs.18105.

18. Jason D. Flatt, Ethan C. Cicero, Krystal R. Kittle, and Mark Brennan-Ing, "Recommendations for Advancing Research with Sexual and Gender Minority Older Adults," *Journals of Gerontology Series B* 77, no. 1 (January 2022): 1–9, https://doi.org/10.1093 /geronb/gbab127.

19. Gilbert Gonzales and Carrie Henning-Smith, "The Affordable Care Act and Health Insurance Coverage for Lesbian, Gay, and Bisexual Adults: Analysis of the Behavioral Risk Factor Surveillance System," *LGBT Health* 4, no. 1 (February 2017): 62–67, https://doi.org/10.1089/lgbt.2016.0023.

20. Carey Candrian and Kristin G. Cloyes, "'She's Dying and I Can't Say We're Married?': End-of-Life Care for LGBT Older Adults,"

Gerontologist 61, no. 8 (November 2021): 1197–201, https://doi
.org/10.1093/geront/gnaa186; and Kelly Haviland, Chasity Burrows Walters, and Susan Newman, "Barriers to Palliative Care
in Sexual and Gender Minority Patients with Cancer: A Scoping Review of the Literature," *Health and Social Care in the Community* 29, no. 2 (March 2021): 305–18, https://doi.org/10.1111
/hsc.13126.

21. National Academies of Sciences, Engineering, and Medicine,
Understanding the Well-Being of LGBTQI+ Populations, edited by
Charlotte J. Patterson, Martín-José Sepúlveda, and Jordyn White
(Washington, DC: The National Academies Press, 2020), https://
doi.org/10.17226/25877; and Jason D. Flatt, Ethan C. Cicero,
Krystal R. Kittle, Mark Brennan-Ing, Joel G. Anderson, Whit-
ney Wharton, and Tonda L. Hughes, "Advancing Gerontological
Health Research with Sexual and Gender Minorities across the
Globe," *Journal of Gerontological Nursing* 48, no. 4 (April 2022):
13–20, https://doi.org/10.3928/00989134-20220304-03.

22. Kate Shaw, Kristina Theis, Shannon Self-Brown, Douglas Roblin,
and Lawrence Barker, "Chronic Disease Disparities by County
Economic Status and Metropolitan Classification, Behavioral
Risk Factor Surveillance System, 2013," *Preventing Chronic Dis-
ease* 13 (September 2016), https://doi.org/10.5888/pcd13.160088;
Gloria L. Krahn, Deborah Klein Walker, and Rosaly Correa-
De-Araujo, "Persons with Disabilities as an Unrecognized Health
Disparity Population," *American Journal of Public Health* 105,
Supplement 2 (April 2015): 198–206, https://doi.org/10.2105
/ajph.2014.302182; Catherine A. Okoro, NaTasha D. Hollis, Alissa
C. Cyrus, and Shannon Griffin-Blake, "Prevalence of Disabilities
and Health Care Access by Disability Status and Type among
Adults—United States, 2016," *Morbidity and Mortality Weekly Re-
port* 67, no. 32 (August 2018): 882–87, https://doi.org/10.15585

/mmwr.mm6732a3; Luisa Kcomt, Kevin M. Gorey, Betty Jo Barrett, and Sean Esteban McCabe, "Healthcare Avoidance Due to Anticipated Discrimination among Transgender People: A Call to Create Trans-Affirmative Environments," *SSM Population Health* 11 (August 2020): 100608, https://doi.org/10.1016/j.ssmph.2020.100608; Sharita Gruberg, Lindsay Mahowald, and John Halpin, *The State of the LGBTQ Community in 2020: A National Public Opinion Study* (Washington, DC: Center for American Progress, 2020), https://www.americanprogress.org/article/state-lgbtq-community-2020/#Ca=10; Jorge Medina-Martínez, Carlos Saus-Ortega, María Montserrat Sánchez-Lorente, Eva María Sosa-Palanca, Pedro García-Martínez, and María Isabel Mármol-López, "Health Inequities in LGBT People and Nursing Interventions to Reduce Them: A Systematic Review," *International Journal of Environmental Research and Public Health* 18, no. 22 (November 2021), https://doi.org/10.3390/ijerph182211801; and Xiaoyong Hu, Tiantian Wang, Duan Huang, Yanli Wang, and Qiong Li, "Impact of Social Class on Health: The Mediating Role of Health Self-Management," *PLoS One* 16, no. 7 (July 2021), https://doi.org/10.1371/journal.pone.0254692.

23. Mary I. O'Connor, "Equity 360: Gender, Race, and Ethnicity—Covid-19 and Preparing for the Next Pandemic," *Clinical Orthopaedics and Related Research* 478, no. 6 (June 2020): 1183–85, https://doi.org/10.1097/corr.0000000000001282; Sanford E. Roberts, "I Can't Breathe—Race, Violence, and Covid-19," *Annals of Surgery* 272, no. 3 (September 2020): 191, https://doi.org/10.1097/sla.0000000000004256; and Alexander Moreno, Salima Belhouari, and Alexane Dussault, "A Systematic Literature Review of the Impact of Covid-19 on the Health of LGBTQI+ Older Adults: Identification of Risk and Protective Health Factors and Development of

a Model of Health and Disease," *Journal of Homosexuality* (February 2023): 1–35, https://doi.org/10.1080/00918369.2023.2169851.

24. American Geriatrics Society Ethics Committee, "American Geriatrics Society Care of Lesbian, Gay, Bisexual, and Transgender Older Adults Position Statement: American Geriatrics Society Ethics Committee," *Journal of the American Geriatrics Society* 63, no. 3 (March 2015): 423–26, https://doi.org/10.1111/jgs.13297; Timothy W. Farrell et al., "Exploring the Intersection of Structural Racism and Ageism in Healthcare," *Journal of the American Geriatrics Society* 70, no. 12 (October 2022): 3366–77, https://doi .org/10.1111/jgs.18105; and Nancy E. Lundebjerg and Annette M. Medina-Walpole, "Future Forward: AGS Initiative Addressing Intersection of Structural Racism and Ageism in Health Care," *Journal of the American Geriatrics Society* 69, no. 4 (April 2021): 892–95, https://doi.org/10.1111/jgs.17053.

25. Stuart M. Lichtman, "Call for Changes in Clinical Trial Reporting of Older Patients with Cancer," *Journal of Clinical Oncology* 30, no. 8 (March 2012): 893–94, https://doi.org/10.1200/jco.2011.41.0696; and Arti Hurria et al., "Designing Therapeutic Clinical Trials for Older and Frail Adults with Cancer: U13 Conference Recommendations," *Journal of Clinical Oncology* 32, no. 24 (August 2014): 2587–94, https://doi.org/10.1200/jco.2013.55.0418.

26. Hurria et al., "Designing Therapeutic Clinical Trials for Older and Frail Adults with Cancer."

27. Harvey M. Chochinov, "The Platinum Rule: A New Standard for Person-Centered Care," *Journal of Palliative Medicine* 25, no. 6 (June 2022): 854–56, https://doi.org/10.1089/jpm.2022.0075.

28. Tony Alessandra and Michael O'Connor, *The Platinum Rule: Discover the Four Basic Business Personalities and How They Can Lead You to Success* (New York: Grand Central Publishing, 1998).

29. Kristine Williams, Clarissa Shaw, Alexandria Lee, Sohyun Kim, Emma Dinneen, Margaret Turk, Ying-Ling Jao, and Wen Liu, "Voicing Ageism in Nursing Home Dementia Care," *Journal of Gerontological Nursing* 43, no. 9 (September 2017): 16–20, https:// doi.org/10.3928/00989134-20170523-02.

30. Howard Giles, Susan Fox, and Elisa Smith, "Patronizing the Elderly: Intergenerational Evaluations," *Research on Language and Social Interaction* 26 (June 1993): 129–49, https://doi.org/10.1207 /s15327973rlsi2602_1.

31. Margaret M. Baltes and Hans-Werner Wahl, "Patterns of Communication in Old Age: The Dependence-Support and Independence-Ignore Script," *Health Communication* 8, no. 3 (July 1996): 217–31, https://doi.org/10.1207/s15327027hc0803_3.

32. Kristine N. Williams, Ruth Herman, Byron Gajewski, and Kristel Wilson, "Elderspeak Communication: Impact on Dementia Care," *American Journal of Alzheimer's Disease & Other Dementias* 24, no. 1 (June 2008): 11–20, https://doi.org/10.11 77/1533317508318472.

33. Ibid.; Judith A. Hall, Debra L. Roter, and Nancy R. Katz, "Meta-Analysis of Correlates of Provider Behavior in Medical Encounters," *Medical Care* 26 (July 1988): 657–75, https://doi .org/10.1097/00005650-198807000-00002; and Jeffrey D. Robinson, "Getting Down to Business Talk, Gaze, and Body Orientation During Openings of Doctor-Patient Consultations," *Human Communication Research* 25, no. 1 (September 1998): 97–123, https://doi.org/10.1111/j.1468-2958.1998.tb00438.x.

34. National Alliance for Caregiving, *Caregiving in a Diverse America: Beginning to Understand the Systemic Challenges Facing Family Caregivers* (Washington, DC: National Alliance for Caregiving, 2023), https://www.caregiving.org/caregiving-in-a

-diverse-america-beginning-to-understand-the-systemic-chal
lenges-facing-family-caregivers/.

35. Centers for Disease Control and Prevention, Alzheimer's Disease and Healthy Aging, *Caregiving among American Indian/ Alaska Native Adults* (Washington, DC: Centers for Disease Control and Prevention, 2019), https://www.cdc.gov/aging/pdf/Clin ical_Preventive_Services_Closing_the_Gap_Report.pdf.

36. National Alliance for Caregiving, *Supporting Diverse Family Caregivers: A Guide for Patient Advocacy Groups* (Washington, DC: National Alliance for Caregiving, 2023), https://www.care giving.org/new-guide-for-patient-advocacy-groups-to-support-diverse-family-caregivers/.

37. Ibid.

38. Hans Wildiers et al., "International Society of Geriatric Oncology Consensus on Geriatric Assessment in Older Patients with Cancer," *Journal of Clinical Oncology* 32, no. 24 (August 2014): 2595–603, https://doi.org/10.1200/jco.2013.54.8347.

39. Matteo Cesari et al., "Added Value of Physical Performance Measures in Predicting Adverse Health-Related Events: Results from the Health, Aging and Body Composition Study," *Journal of the American Geriatrics Society* 57, no. 2 (February 2009): 251–59, https://doi.org/10.1111/j.1532-5415.2008.02126.x; and Stephanie Studenski et al., "Gait Speed and Survival in Older Adults," *Journal of the American Medical Association* 305, no. 1 (January 2011): 50–58, https://doi.org/10.1001/jama.2010.1923.

40. Enrique Soto-Perez-de-Celis, Daneng Li, Yuan Yuan, Yat Ming Lau, and Arti Hurria, "Functional Versus Chronological Age: Geriatric Assessments to Guide Decision Making in Older Patients with Cancer," *Lancet Oncology* 19, no. 6 (June 2018): 305–16, https://doi.org/10.1016/s1470-2045(18)30348-6.

41. Marije E. Hamaker, Anandi H. Schiphorst, Daan ten Bokkel Huinink, Cees Schaar, and Barbara C. van Munster, "The Effect of a Geriatric Evaluation on Treatment Decisions for Older Cancer Patients—A Systematic Review," *Acta Oncologica* 53, no. 3 (March 2014): 289–96, https://doi.org/10.3109/0284186x.2013.840741.

Chapter 5:
Care Is Not One-Size-Fits-All

Save the Last Dance for Me

1. Eli L. Diamond et al., "Prognostic Awareness, Prognostic Communication, and Cognitive Function in Patients with Malignant Glioma," *Neuro-Oncology* 19, no. 11 (October 2017): 1532–41, https://doi.org/10.1093/neuonc/nox117.

2. AARP and the National Alliance for Caregiving, *Cancer Caregiving in the United States: An Intense, Episodic, and Challenging Care Experience* (Washington, DC: National Alliance for Caregiving, 2016), https://www.caregiving.org/wp-content/uploads/2020/05/CancerCaregivingReport_FINAL_June-17-2016.pdf.

3. Andrew Roth, *Managing Prostate Cancer: A Guide for Living Better* (New York: Oxford University Press, 2015).

4. Carma L. Bylund, Richard F. Brown, Philip A. Bialer, Tomer T. Levin, Barbara Lubrano di Ciccone, and David W. Kissane, "Developing and Implementing an Advanced Communication Training Program in Oncology at a Comprehensive Cancer Center," *Journal of Cancer Education* 26, no. 4 (December 2011): 604–11, https://doi.org/10.1007/s13187-011-0226-y; and David W. Kissane, Carma L. Bylund, Smita C. Banerjee, Philip A. Bialer, Tomer T. Levin, Erin K. Maloney, and Thomas A. D'Agostino,

"Communication Skills Training for Oncology Professionals,"
Journal of Clinical Oncology 30, no. 11 (April 2012): 1242–47,
https://doi.org/10.1200/jco.2011.39.6184.

5. Arianne Brinkman-Stoppelenburg, Judith A. C. Rietjens,
and Agnes van der Heide, "The Effects of Advance Care Planning on End-of-Life Care: A Systematic Review," *Palliative
Medicine* 28, no. 8 (September 2014): 1000–1025, https://doi
.org/10.1177/0269216314526272; and Marieke Zwakman, Lea J.
Jabbarian, Johannes J. M. van Delden, Agnes van der Heide, Ida
J. Korfage, Kristian Pollock, Judith A. C. Rietjens, Jane Seymour,
and Marijke C. Kars, "Advance Care Planning: A Systematic Review About Experiences of Patients with a Life-Threatening or
Life-Limiting Illness," *Palliative Medicine* 32, no. 8 (September
2018): 1305–21, https://doi.org/10.1177/0269216318784474.

6. Jennifer S. Temel et al., "Early Palliative Care for Patients with
Metastatic Non-Small-Cell Lung Cancer," *New England Journal of Medicine* 363, no. 8 (August 2010): 733–42, https://doi
.org/10.1056/NEJMoa1000678; Nicholas Dionne-Odom et al.,
"Benefits of Early versus Delayed Palliative Care to Informal
Family Caregivers of Patients with Advanced Cancer: Outcomes
from the Enable III Randomized Controlled Trial," *Journal of
Clinical Oncology* 33, no. 13 (May 2015): 1446–52, https://doi
.org/10.1200/jco.2014.58.7824; and Betty R. Ferrell et al., "Inte-
gration of Palliative Care into Standard Oncology Care: American Society of Clinical Oncology Clinical Practice Guideline
Update," *Journal of Clinical Oncology* 35, no. 1 (January 2017):
96–112, https://doi.org/10.1200/jco.2016.70.1474.

7. Institute of Medicine (US) Committee on Care at the End of
Life, *Approaching Death: Improving Care at the End of Life*, edited
by Marilyn J. Field and Christine K. Cassel (Washington, DC:
National Academics Press, 1997).

8. Alexi A. Wright et al., "Associations between End-of-Life Discussions, Patient Mental Health, Medical Care Near Death, and Caregiver Bereavement Adjustment," *Journal of the American Medical Association* 300, no. 14 (October 2008): 1665–73, https://doi.org/10.1001/jama.300.14.1665; Akiko Akiyama, Kumiko Numata, and Hiroshi Mikami, "Importance of End-of-Life Support to Minimize Caregiver's Regret During Bereavement of the Elderly for Better Subsequent Adaptation to Bereavement," *Archives of Gerontology and Geriatrics* 50, no. 2 (March 2010): 175–78, https://doi.org/10.1016/j.archger.2009.03.006; and Richard Schulz, Kathrin Boerner, Julie Klinger, and Jules Rosen, "Preparedness for Death and Adjustment to Bereavement among Caregivers of Recently Placed Nursing Home Residents," *Journal of Palliative Medicine* 18, no. 2 (February 2015): 127–33, https://doi.org/10.1089/jpm.2014.0309.

9. Kelly Haviland, Chasity Burrows Walters, and Susan Newman, "Barriers to Palliative Care in Sexual and Gender Minority Patients with Cancer: A Scoping Review of the Literature," *Health and Social Care in the Community* 29, no. 2 (March 2021): 305–18, https://doi.org/10.1111/hsc.13126.

10. Nina Barrett and Dorothy Wholihan, "Providing Palliative Care to LGBTQ Patients," *Nursing Clinics of North America* 51, no. 3 (September 2016): 501–11, https://doi.org/10.1016/j.cnur.2016.05.001; and Mark Hughes and Colleen Cartwright, "Lesbian, Gay, Bisexual and Transgender People's Attitudes to End-of-Life Decision-Making and Advance Care Planning," *Australasian Journal on Ageing* 34, Supplement 2 (October 2015): 39–43, https://doi.org/10.1111/ajag.12268.

11. Carey Candrian and Kristin G. Cloyes, "'She's Dying and I Can't Say We're Married?': End-of-Life Care for LGBT Older Adults," *Gerontologist* 61, no. 8 (November 2021): 1197–201, https://doi.org/10.1093/geront/gnaa186.

12. William E. Rosa, Smita C. Banerjee, and Shail Maingi, "Family Caregiver Inclusion Is Not a Level Playing Field: Toward Equity for the Chosen Families of Sexual and Gender Minority Patients," *Palliative Care and Social Practice* 16 (April 2022): 2632352422 1092459, https://doi.org/10.1177/26323524221092459.

13. Kenneth J. Doka, *Disenfranchised Grief: Recognizing Hidden Sorrow* (Lanham, MD: Lexington Books, 1989).

14. Katherine Bristowe et al., "LGBT+ Partner Bereavement and Appraisal of the Acceptance-Disclosure Model of LGBT+ Bereavement: A Qualitative Interview Study," *Palliative Medicine* 37, no. 2 (February 2023): 221–34, https://doi.org/10.1177/02692163221138620.

15. Tomer T. Levin, Beatriz Moreno, William Silvester, and David W. Kissane, "End-of-Life Communication in the Intensive Care Unit," *General Hospital Psychiatry* 32, no. 4 (July 2010): 433–42, https://doi.org/10.1016/j.genhosppsych.2010.04.007; Daren K. Heyland et al., "Failure to Engage Hospitalized Elderly Patients and Their Families in Advance Care Planning," *JAMA Internal Medicine* 173, no. 9 (May 2013): 778–87, https://doi.org/10.1001/jamainternmed.2013.180; and John J. You, Robert A. Fowler, and Daren K. Heyland, "Just Ask: Discussing Goals of Care with Patients in Hospital with Serious Illness," *Canadian Medical Association Journal* 186, no. 6 (April 2014): 425–32, https://doi.org/10.1503/cmaj.121274.

16. Joseph J. Fins, *Rights Come to Mind: Brain Injury, Ethics, and the Struggle for Consciousness* (Cambridge, MA: Cambridge University Press, 2015).

17. Harvey M. Chochinov, "The Platinum Rule: A New Standard for Person-Centered Care," *Journal of Palliative Medicine* 25, no. 6 (June 2022): 854–56, https://doi.org/10.1089/jpm.2022.0075.

Chapter 6:
The Caregiving House of Cards

A Little Bit of Everything

1. Kate Washington, *Already Toast: Caregiving and Burnout in America* (Boston: Beacon Press, 2021).
2. Howard J. Markman, Scott M. Stanley, and Susan L. Blumberg, *Fighting for Your Marriage: A Deluxe Revised Edition of the Classic Best-Seller for Enhancing Marriage and Preventing Divorce* (San Francisco: Jossey-Bass, 2010).

Chapter 7: Team Sports

Where the Boys Are

1. PHI, *Direct Care Workers in the United States: Key Facts* (New York: PHI, 2022), https://www.phinational.org/resource/direct-care-workers-in-the-united-states-key-facts-3/.
2. Stephen Campbell, Angelina Del Rio Drake, Robert Espinoza, and Kezia Scales, *Caring for the Future: The Power and Potential of America's Direct Care Workforce* (New York: PHI, 2021), http://www.phinational.org/caringforthefuture/.
3. Bureau of Labor Statistics, *Standard Occupational Classification*, accessed December 7, 2022, https://www.bls.gov/soc/2018/home.htm.
4. PHI, *Direct Care Workers in the United States*.
5. Deirdre McCaughey, Gwen McGhan, Jungyoon Kim, Diane Brannon, Hannes Leroy, and Rita Jablonski, "Workforce Impli-

cations of Injury among Home Health Workers: Evidence from the National Home Health Aide Survey," *Gerontologist* 52, no. 4 (August 2012): 493–505, https://doi.org/10.1093/geront/gnr133; and Joanne Spetz, Robyn I. Stone, Susan A. Chapman, and Natasha Bryant, "Home and Community-Based Workforce for Patients with Serious Illness Requires Support to Meet Growing Needs," *Health Affairs* 38, no. 6 (June 2019): 902–9, https://doi .org/10.1377/hlthaff.2019.00021.

6. Social Security Agency, *Fact Sheet: Social Security*, accessed December 7, 2022, https://www.ssa.gov/news/press/factsheets/basic fact-alt.pdf.

7. LawHelp.org, "Find Free Legal Help and Information about Your Legal Rights from Nonprofit Legal Aid Providers in Your State," Lawhelp.org, Pro Bono Net, accessed April 18, 2023, https://www.lawhelp.org/.

8. Nursing Home Law Center, "For an Individual, How Much Does It Cost to Treat Bed Sores?" accessed December 9, 2022, https://www.nursinghomelawcenter.org/for-an-individual-how -much-does-it-cost-to-treat-bed-sores.html.

9. Homer, *The Odyssey*, translated by Robert Fagles (London: Penguin Classics, 1999).

10. AARP and the National Alliance for Caregiving, *Cancer Caregiving in the United States: An Intense, Episodic, and Challenging Care Experience* (Washington, DC: National Alliance for Caregiving, 2016), https://www.caregiving.org/wp-content/uploads /2020/05/CancerCaregivingReport_FINAL_June-17-2016.pdf.

Chapter 8: Surfing the Waves of Grief

Stairway to Heaven

1. Therese A. Rando, *Loss and Anticipatory Grief* (Marlborough, MA: Lexington Books, 1986).
2. Alexandra Coelho, Maja de Brito, and Antonio Barbosa, "Caregiver Anticipatory Grief: Phenomenology, Assessment and Clinical Interventions," *Current Opinion in Supportive and Palliative Care* 12, no. 1 (March 2018): 52–57, https://doi.org/10.1097/spc.0000000000000321.
3. Jonathan Singer, Kailey E. Roberts, Elisabeth McLean, Carol Fadalla, Taylor Coats, Madeline Rogers, Madeline K. Wilson, Kendra Godwin, and Wendy G. Lichtenthal, "An Examination and Proposed Definitions of Family Members' Grief Prior to the Death of Individuals with a Life-Limiting Illness: A Systematic Review," *Palliative Medicine* 36, no. 4 (April 2022): 581–608, https://doi.org/10.1177/02692163221074540.
4. Noam Schneck, Tao Tu, Stefan Haufe, George A. Bonanno, Hanga Galfavy, Kevin N. Ochsner, J. John Mann, and Paul Sajda, "Ongoing Monitoring of Mindwandering in Avoidant Grief through Cortico-Basal-Ganglia Interactions," *Social Cognitive and Affective Neuroscience* 14, no. 2 (February 2019): 163–72, https://doi.org/10.1093/scan/nsy114.
5. Nancy Stein, Susan Folkman, Tom Trabasso, and Anne Richards, "Appraisal and Goal Processes as Predictors of Psychological Well-Being in Bereaved Caregivers," *Journal of Personality and Social Psychology* 72 (April 1997): 872–84, https://doi.org/10.1037/0022-3514.72.4.872.

6. Kailey Roberts, Jimmie Holland, Holly G. Prigerson, Corinne Sweeney, Geoffrey Corner, William Breitbart, and Wendy G. Lichtenthal, "Development of the Bereavement Risk Inventory and Screening Questionnaire (BRISQ): Item Generation and Expert Panel Feedback," *Palliative and Supportive Care* 15, no. 1 (February 2017): 57–66, https://doi.org/10.1017 /s1478951516000626.

7. American Psychiatric Association, *Diagnostic and Statistical Manual of Mental Disorders (DSM-5-TR)* (Washington, DC: American Psychiatric Publishing, 2022).

8. M. Katherine Shear, "Grief Is a Form of Love," in Robert A. Neimeyer, ed., *Techniques of Grief Therapy: Assessment and Intervention* (New York: Routledge/Taylor and Francis Group, 2016), 14–18.

9. Judith L. M. McCoyd, Jeanne Koller, and Carolyn Ambler Walter, *Grief and Loss Across the Lifespan: A Biopsychosocial Perspective* (New York: Springer, 2021).

10. Grace H. Christ, George Bonanno, Ruth Malkinson, and Simon Rubin, "Bereavement Experiences After the Death of a Child," in Marilyn J. Field and Richard E. Behrman, eds., *When Children Die: Improving Palliative and End-of-Life Care for Children and Their Families* (Washington, DC: National Academies Press, 2003).

11. Wendy G. Lichtenthal and William Breitbart, "The Central Role of Meaning in Adjustment to the Loss of a Child to Cancer: Implications for the Development of Meaning-Centered Grief Therapy," *Current Opinion in Supportive and Palliative Care* 9, no. 1 (March 2015): 46–51, https://doi.org/10.1097 /spc.0000000000000117; Wendy G. Lichtenthal, Joseph M. Currier, Robert A. Neimeyer, and Nancy J. Keesee, "Sense and Sig-

nificance: A Mixed Methods Examination of Meaning Making after the Loss of One's Child," *Journal of Clinical Psychology* 66, no. 7 (July 2010): 791–812, https://doi.org/10.1002/jclp.20700; and Wendy G. Lichtenthal et al., "Regret and Unfinished Business in Parents Bereaved by Cancer: A Mixed Methods Study," *Palliative Medicine* 34, no. 3 (March 2020): 367–77, https://doi.org/10.1177/0269216319900301.

12. US Department of Labor, Wage and Hour Division, "Family and Medical Leave Act," accessed December 7, 2022, https://www.dol.gov/agencies/whd/fmla.

Chapter 9:
Finding Meaning in Caregiving

The Goin's Great

1. William S. Breitbart, ed., *Meaning-Centered Psychotherapy in the Cancer Setting: Finding Meaning and Hope in the Face of Suffering* (New York: Oxford University Press, 2017).
2. Viktor Frankl, *Man's Search for Meaning* (Boston: Beacon Press, 2006).
3. Viktor Frankl, *Man's Search for Ultimate Meaning* (New York: Plenum, 1975/1997).
4. Breitbart, ed., *Meaning-Centered Psychotherapy in the Cancer Setting*.
5. Richard Lazarus and Susan Folkman, *Stress, Appraisal, and Coping* (New York: Springer, 1984).
6. Susan Folkman, Margaret A. Chesney, and Anne Christopher-Richards, "Stress and Coping in Caregiving Partners of Men with AIDS," *Psychiatric Clinics of North America* 17 (March 1994): 35–53, https://doi.org/10.1016/S0193-953X(18)30129-1.

7. Crystal L. Park, "Meaning Making in the Context of Disasters," *Journal of Clinical Psychology* 72, no. 12 (December 2016): 1234–46, https://doi.org/https://doi.org/10.1002/jclp.22270.

8. Anna Elderton, Alexis Berry, and Carmen Chan, "A Systematic Review of Posttraumatic Growth in Survivors of Interpersonal Violence in Adulthood," *Trauma Violence & Abuse* 18, no. 2 (April 2017): 223–36, https://doi.org/10.1177/1524838015611672.

9. Cengiz Kılıç, Katherine M. Magruder, and Mehmet M. Koryürek, "Does Trauma Type Relate to Posttraumatic Growth after War? A Pilot Study of Young Iraqi War Survivors Living in Turkey," *Transcultural Psychiatry* 53, no. 1 (February 2016): 110–23, https://doi.org/10.1177/1363461515612963.

10. Susan Cadell, "The Sun Always Comes Out After It Rains: Understanding Posttraumatic Growth in HIV Caregivers," *Health and Social Work* 32, no. 3 (August 2007): 169–76, https://doi.org/10.1093/hsw/32.3.169; Youngmee Kim, Richard Schulz, and Charles S. Carver, "Benefit Finding in the Cancer Caregiving Experience," *Psychosomatic Medicine* 69, no. 3 (April 2007): 283–91, https://doi.org/10.1097/PSY.0b013e3180417cf4; Tony Cassidy, "Benefit Finding through Caring: The Cancer Caregiver Experience," *Psychology and Health* 28, no. 3 (July 2012): 250–66, https://doi.org/10.1080/08870446.2012.717623; Claudia Cormio, Francesca Romito, Giovanna Viscanti, Marina Turaccio, Vito Lorusso, and Vittorio Mattioli, "Psychological Well-Being and Posttraumatic Growth in Caregivers of Cancer Patients," *Frontiers in Psychology* 5 (November 2014), https://doi.org/10.3389/fpsyg.2014.01342; and Charles Brand, Lorna Barry, and Stephen Gallagher, "Social Support Mediates the Association between Benefit Finding and Quality of Life in Caregivers," *Journal of Health Psychology* 21, no. 6 (June 2016): 1126–36, https://doi.org/10.1177/1359105314547244.

11. Carole A. Cohen, Angela Colantonio, and Lee Vernich, "Positive Aspects of Caregiving: Rounding out the Caregiver Experience," *International Journal of Geriatric Psychiatry* 17, no. 2 (February 2002): 184–88, https://doi.org/10.1002/gps.561; and William E. Haley, Laurie A. LaMonde, Beth Han, Allison M. Burton, and Ronald Schonwetter, "Predictors of Depression and Life Satisfaction among Spousal Caregivers in Hospice: Application of a Stress Process Model," *Journal of Palliative Medicine* 6, no. 2 (April 2003): 215–24, https://doi.org/10.1089/109662103764978461.

12. Haley et al., "Predictors of Depression and Life Satisfaction"; Viktor Frankl, *Man's Search for Meaning: An Introduction to Logotherapy* (New York: Washington Square Press, 1963); Youngmee Kim, Frank Baker, and Rachel L. Spillers, "Cancer Caregivers' Quality of Life: Effects of Gender, Relationship, and Appraisal," *Journal of Pain and Symptom Management* 34, no. 3 (September 2007): 294–304, https://doi.org/10.1016/j.jpainsymman.2006.11.012; and Betty J. Kramer, "Gain in the Caregiving Experience: Where Are We? What Next?" *Gerontologist* 37, no. 2 (April 1997): 218–32, https://doi.org/10.1093/geront/37.2.218.

13. Avinash Thombre, Allen C. Sherman, and Stephanie Simonton, "Religious Coping and Posttraumatic Growth among Family Caregivers of Cancer Patients in India," *Journal of Psychosocial Oncology* 28, no. 2 (February 2010): 173–88, https://doi.org/10.1080/07347330903570537.

14. Peter Hudson, "Positive Aspects and Challenges Associated with Caring for a Dying Relative at Home," *International Journal of Palliative Nursing* 10, no. 2 (February 2004): 58–65, https://doi.org/10.12968/ijpn.2004.10.2.12454.

15. Mariko Asai, Maiko Fujimori, Nobuya Akizuki, Masatoshi Inagaki, Yutaka Matsui, and Yosuke Uchitomi, "Psychological States

and Coping Strategies after Bereavement among the Spouses of Cancer Patients: A Qualitative Study," *Psycho-Oncology* 19, no. 1 (January 2010): 38–45, https://doi.org/10.1002/pon.1444; and Monika Brandstätter, Monika Kögler, Urs Baumann, Veronika Fensterer, Helmut Küchenhoff, Gian Domenico Borasio, and Martin Johannes Fegg, "Experience of Meaning in Life in Bereaved Informal Caregivers of Palliative Care Patients," *Supportive Care in Cancer* 22, no. 5 (May 2014): 1391–99, https://doi.org/10.1007/s00520-013-2099-6.

16. Allison J. Applebaum, Raymond E. Baser, Kailey E. Roberts, Kathleen Lynch, Rebecca Gebert, William S. Breitbart, and Eli L. Diamond, "Meaning-Centered Psychotherapy for Cancer Caregivers: A Pilot Trial among Caregivers of Patients with Glioblastoma Multiforme," *Translational Behavioral Medicine* 12, no. 8 (August 2022): 841–52, https://doi.org/10.1093/tbm/ibac043; Allison J. Applebaum et al., "A Qualitative Exploration of the Feasibility and Acceptability of Meaning-Centered Psychotherapy for Cancer Caregivers," *Palliative and Supportive Care* 20, no. 5 (October 2022): 623–29, https://doi.org/10.1017/s1478951521002030; and Allison J. Applebaum, Kara L. Buda, Elizabeth Schofield, Maria Farberov, Nicole D. Teitelbaum, Katherine Evans, Rebecca Cowens-Alvarado, and Rachel S. Cannady, "Exploring the Cancer Caregiver's Journey through Web-Based Meaning-Centered Psychotherapy," *Psycho-Oncology* 27, no. 3 (March 2018): 847–56, https://doi.org/10.1002/pon.4583.

17. Allison J. Applebaum, "Meaning-Centered Psychotherapy for Cancer Caregivers," in Allison J. Applebaum, ed., *Cancer Caregivers* (New York: Oxford University Press, 2019), 237–53.

18. Rollo May, *The Courage to Create* (New York: Norton, 1994).

19. Applebaum, "Meaning-Centered Psychotherapy for Cancer Caregivers."

20. Arthur Kleinman, *The Soul of Care: The Moral Education of a Husband and a Doctor* (London: Penguin Books Ltd, 2020), 170.

Chapter 10:
Stepping into the Spotlight

Stand By Me

1. "State Law to Help Family Caregivers," AARP, 2014, https://www.aarp.org/politics-society/advocacy/caregiving-advocacy/info-2014/aarp-creates-model-state-bill.html; and Joan M. Griffin et al., "Improving Transitions in Care for Patients and Family Caregivers Living in Rural and Underserved Areas: The Caregiver Advise, Record, Enable (Care) Act," *Journal of Aging and Social Policy* (February 2022): 1–8, https://doi.org/10.1080/08959420.2022.2029272.

2. Susan C. Reinhard, Selena Caldera, Ari Houser, and Rita B. Choula, *Valuing the Invaluable: 2023 Update Strengthening Supports for Family Caregivers* (Washington, DC: AARP Public Policy Institute, 2023), https://doi.org/10.26419/ppi.00082.006.

3. Family Caregiver Alliance, *Caregiver Statistics: Health, Technology, and Caregiving Resources* (San Francisco: Family Caregiver Alliance, 2016), https://www.caregiver.org/resource/caregiver-statistics-health-technology-and-caregiving-resources/.

4. Office of the Law Revision Council, "US Code Chapter 28—Family and Medical Leave," accessed December 7, 2022, https://uscode.house.gov/view.xhtml?path=/prelim@title29/chapter28&edition=prelim.

5. US Department of Labor, Wage and Hour Division, "FMLA Frequently Asked Questions," accessed November 11, 2022, https://www.dol.gov/agencies/whd/fmla/faq.

6. Allison J. Applebaum, "Meaning-Centered Psychotherapy for Cancer Caregivers," in Allison J. Applebaum, ed., *Cancer Caregivers* (New York: Oxford University Press, 2019), 237–53.

7. *Family Caregiving Issues and the National Family Caregiver Support Program, Before the Senate Special Committee on Aging*, statement of former First Lady Rosalynn Carter, 2011.

INDEX

Note: Italic page numbers refer to tables and figures.

caregivers *(cont.)*
  as case managers, 151, 157–60
  categories of caregiving tasks,
    32–33
  chosen family members as,
    31, 139
  compassion fatigue of,
    254–55
  complementary strengths of,
    55
  defining qualities of, 30–31
  delegation of tasks and,
    32–33, 55–56, 57
  difficult family relationships
    and, 162–67, 257
  on discharge as anxiety-
    provoking experience,
    154–55, 245
  discrimination against, 90–91,
    106–11
  duties of, 31–39
  emotional and psychological
    needs of, 16
  existential distress of, 8
  as extension of healthcare
    team, 13, 243, 245, 256,
    260, 261
  as family mediators, 151,
    160–67, 257
  fear of death of loved one
    and, 6, 77–78
  financial demands of
    caregiving and, 6, 11, 33,
    36, 49, 50, 56, 57, 66, 150,
    158, 159, 168

  functional age of patient
    advocated by, 111–12
  goals of life and, 119
  healthcare proxy and, 124–25
  health conditions of, 36, 251,
    254
  hours per week of care
    provided by, 31–32
  identification of, 253–54, 265
  impact on quality of care, 5,
    9, 13, 15, 108
  incremental nature of
    caregiving and, 29
  as keeper of patient's legacy,
    13, 14, 28, 208, 266
  length of caregiving, 31–32
  life goals of, 168
  liminal space experienced by,
    8–9
  Meaning-Centered
    Psychotherapy for, 225
  medical and nursing tasks of,
    33, 66, 150, 151–57
  mental health of, 11, 245
  non-choice choices of, 55
  patient's goals of care and,
    120–22
  physical health of, 11
  planning for present and
    future, 6, 7, 8–9, 67
  population of, 31
  positive and negative
    emotions experienced by,
    9, 10
  providing care for individuals

conversations with, 93–94,
100
Medicare, 95, 180–81
medication management, 249
memorial services, 203–4, 211,
266
Memorial Sloan Kettering
Cancer Center, 16, 129
mental health
assessment for mental health
concerns in grief, 202
discrimination associated
with poor health
outcomes and, 95
emotional support and,
247–51
good death and, 135
palliative care and, 134
risk factors for, 200–201
metacognitions, 66, 77, 83
middle-age adult caregivers, 36,
37
mindful living, capacity for, 81
mindfulness-based practices
cognitive restructuring and,
70–71, 74–81, 85
coping strategies and, 60, 64,
66–69, 77–78, 79, 80–81
letting go and, 82–85
rumination and, 63–65, 68,
76–77
sitting with emotions and, 78
stress-management strategies
and, 85–88, 89

uncertainty and, 66–67, 84, 85
unhelpful thought patterns
and, 71, 72–73, 74
worry and, 63–69
See also uncertainty
mind reading, 107–8
mourner's Kaddish, 203–4

National Alliance for
Caregiving, 30–31, 58, 106
nature, transcendence through, 2
negative self-talk, 76, 78
networks of silence, 127, 132
New York Legal Assistance
Group (NYLAG), 182
New York Public Library for the
Performing Arts, 19, 145
Nietzsche, Friedrich, 219
911 calls, caregivers' storytelling
role in, 14, 22
no evidence of disease (NED),
52, 65
non-Hodgkin's lymphoma, 67
Notov, Ida, 226–27
nurses
caregivers' storytelling role
and, 14–15, 17
visiting nurses, 33, 152, 246
nursing home care, 158, 171,
173, 181

old age, concept of, 93
older adult caregivers, 36, 37
one-on-one counseling, 248

ABOUT THE AUTHOR

Allison J. Applebaum, PhD, is a clinical psychologist specializing in psycho-oncology, the field devoted to supporting the mental health of all individuals affected by cancer. She is an associate attending psychologist in the Department of Psychiatry and Behavioral Sciences at Memorial Sloan Kettering Cancer Center (MSK), and an associate professor of psychology in psychiatry at Weill Cornell Medicine in New York City. Dr. Applebaum is the founding director of the Caregivers Clinic at MSK. The Caregivers Clinic is the first of its kind and provides targeted psychosocial care to caregivers—family members and friends—of patients receiving cancer care at MSK.